End of Life Choices for Cancer Patients

End of Life Choices for
Cancer Patients

EBN HEALTH

OXFORD, UK

TK

Contents

Contributors

Professor Michael I. Bennett, Head, Academic Unit of Palliative Care, Leeds Institute of Health Sciences, University of Leeds, Leeds, UK

Dr Isra Black, Lecturer in Law, York Law School, University of York, York, UK

Dr Ruth E. Board, Consultant in Medical Oncology, Rosemere Cancer Centre, Royal Preston Hospital, Lancashire Teaching Hospitals NHS Foundation Trust, Preston, UK

Professor Rob George, Medical Director, St Christopher's Hospice, London, UK; Department of Palliative Care, Policy and Rehabilitation, King's College London, London, UK

Professor Penney Lewis, Co-Director, Centre of Medical Law and Ethics, Dickson Poon School of Law, King's College London, London, UK

Dr Madeline Li, Psychiatrist, Department of Supportive Care, Princess Margaret Cancer Centre, University Health Network, Toronto, ON, Canada

Dr Andrew Page, NIHR Academic Clinical Fellow in Palliative Medicine, Academic Unit of Palliative Care, Leeds Institute of Health Sciences, University of Leeds, Leeds, UK

Dr Amy Proffitt, Deputy Medical Director and Consultant in Palliative Medicine, St Christopher's Hospice, London, UK

Dr Gary Rodin, Head, Department of Supportive Care, Princess Margaret Cancer Centre, University Health Network, Toronto, ON, Canada

Professor Peter Selby, Professor of Cancer Medicine, University of Leeds, Leeds, UK; President, Association of Cancer Physicians

Dr Gilla Shapiro, Postdoctoral Fellow, Department of Supportive Care, Princess Margaret Cancer Centre, University Health Network, Toronto, ON, Canada

Professor John Wagstaff, Professor of Medical Oncology, College of Medicine, Swansea University, Swansea, UK; Director, South West Wales Cancer Research Institute, Swansea, UK

Dr Joshua Wales, Physician, Temmy Latner Centre for Palliative Care, Sinai Health System, University of Toronto, Toronto, ON, Canada

Chapter 1: Introduction and Summary

Ruth E. Board, Michael I. Bennett, Penney Lewis, Peter Selby

There have been impressive improvements in the diagnosis and treatment of cancer in recent decades. In economically advantaged countries with well-developed healthcare systems, over 50% of all cancer patients achieve long-term survival and are probably cured.[1] This much-improved outcome may be compared with a figure of only 25% in the latter half of the 20th century in these countries.[1] Not only has survival improved radically for cancer patients but also there has been an increasing focus on the quality of patients) lives, on improving the patient experience of care and on developing effective support for the very many cancer survivors.[1]

Major scientific and technological developments are continuing and the practice of oncology is becoming more precise and with more accurate patient selection for appropriate treatment.[2] In addition to surgery, radiotherapy and chemotherapy, there are important developing and successful new modalities of treatment, including immunotherapy[3] and interventions that can destroy tumours using heat, cold, electricity, radio waves and ultrasound without major surgical procedures. There still remain many challenges to be addressed if we are to continue to improve cancer therapy and its outcome. Not only must we vigorously pursue the scientific and technical advances that are providing improvements but we must also ensure that care for cancer patients is well organized with timely access to the appropriate diagnosis and treatment.[1] We must provide high-quality and timely support for patients who have acute medical problems and complications from cancer.[4] We must recognize that cancer is most commonly a disease of elderly people and adjust our approaches to make them feasible and acceptable for all patients.[5]

Despite the progress outlined above, a substantial number of cancer patients will still ultimately die of their disease. For many this will follow periods of successful treatment that resulted in good remissions and good quality of life. However, when patients relapse, the disease may become resistant to available treatment. Helping patients to make the right choices about their care towards the end of their lives is one of the greatest and most challenging responsibilities of all healthcare professionals. Choosing treatments to relieve symptoms is often difficult. Decisions on the continuation of specific anticancer treatments to prolong life or relieve symptoms are complex and uncertain and depend greatly on our ability to elicit the patient's needs and preferences. The involvement of partners, family and friends is often important but must be achieved without overshadowing the patient's own views. Oncology and palliative care professionals from many disciplines work together in teams in order to provide the best possible help for their patients.

There is currently an added dimension that we feel needs to be considered. Legal change on the provision of assisted dying by healthcare professionals has occurred in a substantial number of jurisdictions. There is some pressure for change in UK law and some UK patients travel to other jurisdictions to access assisted dying.

The Association of Cancer Physicians) workshop

The workshop of the Association of Cancer Physicians (ACP) 'End of life choices for cancer patients: an international perspective) was held in Leeds in May 2019 and brought together colleagues from oncology disciplines, palliative care, law, nursing and professions allied to medicine. The goals were to allow an exchange of information through formal presentations and discussion:

- to better inform ACP members and the wider community about developments in choices in end of life care for cancer patients in the UK and internationally;
- to be better able to answer questions from patients and respond to their requests, including questions about and requests for assisted dying in countries outside the UK;
- to have a balanced and well-informed dialogue about choices available to patients in the UK and internationally, without developing a formal ACP position on change in UK law;
- to provide a basis of information for future educational activities.

Definitions

The topic of assisted dying involves a wide range of terms and definitions that are constantly changing. In the ACP workshop and publication we have used the terminologies shown in the Box 1.1 below.

Box 1.1 Definitions.

- Euthanasia: An intervention undertaken with the intention of ending a life to relieve suffering. In the Dutch and Belgian contexts, the term euthanasia refers only to the termination of life upon request.

Some common (and often confusing) modifiers of euthanasia are:
  - He has Active: A deliberate intervention to end life.
  - Passive: Withdrawal/withholding of life-sustaining treatment.
  - Voluntary: At the request of the person killed.
  - Involuntary: In the absence of a request by the person killed, although that person is competent.
  - Non-voluntary: In the absence of a request by the person killed, when that person is not competent and has not made an advance request for euthanasia.
- Assisted suicide: Any act that intentionally helps another person to commit suicide, for example by providing him or her with the means to do so. In the Netherlands, assisted suicide is often included in the term euthanasia. Legal regimes often permit only physician-assisted suicide.
- Assisted dying: (Voluntary, active) euthanasia and assisted suicide.
- Physician-assisted death: This includes physician-administered voluntary euthanasia and physician-assisted suicide.
- Medical assistance in dying (MAID): Used most recently in Canada and includes physician-assisted suicide and clinician-administered voluntary euthanasia.

The legal debate on assisted dying in the UK

As we will discuss in Chapters 3 and 4, assisted dying, whether in the form of assisted suicide or voluntary euthanasia, is illegal in the UK in all jurisdictions. However, in any year several dozen people from the UK travel abroad for assistance in suicide or euthanasia. Doubts and uncertainties about the role of family members in helping them do so cause considerable anxiety. However, in February 2010, the Director of Public Prosecutions set out the factors to be considered when deciding whether a prosecution in an assisted suicide case is in the public interest (the policy is discussed in Chapter 4). The policy suggests that it is unlikely to be in the public interest for a loved one who has provided assistance to be prosecuted if the person who travelled to another jurisdiction for assistance with suicide had reached a voluntary, clear, settled and informed decision to do so, and the loved one who had helped them was motivated by compassion.

In the UK there have been attempts to change the law on assisted dying since 1931, when a voluntary euthanasia bill was proposed. The Voluntary Euthanasia Society was formed in 1935. This society is now known as Dignity in Dying. Another attempt at legal reform was made in 1936, and again in the House of Lords in 1969 and 1976. An assisted dying bill was introduced into the Commons in 1997 but was defeated. Lord Joffe introduced bills between 2003 and 2006 without success. Lord Falconer introduced an assisted dying bill into the House of Lords in 2014, proposing that patients with a life expectancy of less than 6 months should have the choice of a medically assisted death, but it did not succeed. In 2015, the MP Rob Marris brought forward a private member's bill proposing assisted suicide, which was substantially based on Lord Falconer's proposals. The bill was defeated in the House of Commons in September 2015. In 2016, Lord Hayward introduced an assisted dying bill in the Lords, but it did not progress.

The law in Scotland is of course different from the law of England and Wales. Most recently, in 2015, a proposal to change the law was defeated in the Scottish parliament. In February 2019, a group was formed in the Scottish parliament seeking to attempt to reform assisted dying law in Scotland. There have been no recent efforts to change the law in Northern Ireland.

Among Crown dependencies and overseas territories, the Falkland Islands) representatives voted in July 2018 to allow assisted dying for the terminally ill subject to safeguards, in principle indicating a willingness to change their law if the UK did so. On the other hand, also in 2018, representatives in Guernsey voted against a change in the law to allow access to assisted dying. Currently there is an ongoing debate in Jersey, in response to a petition, and Jersey's health minister has called for laws banning assisted dying to be reviewed.

Among Commonwealth countries, Canada has recently changed its law following a successful constitutional challenge (discussed in Chapter 5). The Australian state of Victoria's Voluntary Assisted Dying Act came into effect on 19 June 2019.[6] A similar law in Western Australia was passed by the state legislature in December 2019 and is likely to come into force in 2021.[7] The New Zealand parliament has recently debated and approved an approach to the provision of assisted dying in New Zealand and is placing its proposed detailed legislation before the citizens of New Zealand in a referendum.[8] In Chapters 3 and 5 we will describe the approaches to choices at the end of life that have been developed in other countries and in particular focus on the recent experience in Canada over the last 3 years. The international situation remains dynamic.

Against such a complex background we have sought in our workshop and this publication to provide an informative and balanced review of international experience and current UK relevant healthcare practice for healthcare professionals and those considering a change in the law in the UK.

Summary of the workshop and this edited collection

Dr Ruth Board gave an oncology and patient-centred overview of the choices faced by cancer patients, which is presented in Chapter 2. She introduced the debate on assisted dying and reported recent survey evidence of the attitudes of UK clinicians to possible changes in legislation. The recent survey evidence from the Royal College of Physicians and the Royal College of Radiologists indicates a change in attitudes among oncologists. The professionals surveyed are, according to these data, broadly neutral in their attitude to a change in legislation governing choices at the end of life. However, importantly, as discussed in more detail by Professor Rob George and Dr Amy Proffitt in Chapter 7, palliative care physicians are broadly against any change in UK law. Professor John Wagstaff described his experience as a medical oncologist working in the Netherlands during the early years of the introduction of lawful assisted dying for patients.

There was a consensus in the workshop that the decisions about changing legislation should be influenced most by social, legal and political opinion and should not be heavily influenced by those of healthcare professionals. The views of healthcare professionals are important, not because they should guide or shape public opinion but because these professionals are closely involved in the provision of good-quality care for patients at the end of life and will continue to be so. Any legislative change will have an impact on the patterns and quality of clinical practice and communication with patients.

Professor Penney Lewis and Dr Isra Black laid out for clinical colleagues the law that governs choices at the end of life in jurisdictions around the world. These are presented in Chapters 3 and 4. How the law was changed in the Netherlands, Belgium, Luxembourg, Switzerland, nine US states, Columbia and, more recently, Canada was described for these jurisdictions, which have in recent decades changed their law to permit, variously, assisted suicide and/or euthanasia. Important definitions were set out (summarized in Box 1.1). Professor Lewis summarized features of permissive assisted dying regimes, their oversight and reporting and the frequency of different end of life decisions. Dr Black described the law as it applies in England and Wales and illustrated how the law applied to current practice in the care of cancer patients covering refusal of life-prolonging treatments, advance decisions, stopping eating and drinking, withholding or withdrawing life-prolonging treatment, euthanasia and assisted suicide.

The most recent experience of a significant change in the choices available to patients at the end of life comes from Canada. This was explained to us by Professor Gary Rodin at the workshop and together with Dr Gilla Shapiro, Dr Joshua Wales and Dr Madeline Li, he summarises his presentation in Chapter 5. The law in Canada changed when the Supreme Court of Canada ruled that the criminal prohibition of assisted suicide was unconstitutional. Professor Rodin described the experience of implementing MAID across Canada in the last 3 years. Broadly, Professor Rodin and his colleagues concluded that the introduction of MAID has been possible, has affected a relatively small proportion of patients, and while creating debate and some tension within healthcare circles has not been associated with any evidence of deterioration in the quality of care in a country with good access to palliative care. Further developments that will address important subgroups, including older children and some vulnerable adults, are under discussion in Canada.

Professor Michael Bennett summarized palliative care services in the UK and what they are achieving for patients. He and Dr Andrew Page present their summary in Chapter 6. Professor Bennett described how palliative care in the UK was among the best in the world and evidence showed its efficacy in many cases. However, the duration of palliative care for cancer patients remained relatively short and there was evidence of inequitable access. Professor Rob George described the rational basis of palliative care and end of life choices and he and Dr Amy Proffitt present this and the views of palliative care professionals in Chapter 7. They agreed that decisions about change in the law must be seen as a wide social, legal and political development but felt professionals should express their views on how changes could be implemented while ensuring we continued to maintain the best in healthcare services. Their conclusion, importantly, was that if there were to be changes in the law then implementation of assisted suicide or euthanasia should be kept separate from the provision of palliative care for cancer patients and other patients at the end of life.

In Chapter 8, the editors draw out some broad conclusions from the discussions in the workshop and from the contributions of their colleagues.

References

1   Velikova G, Fallowfield L, Younger J, et al., eds. Problem solving in patient-centred and integrated cancer care. Oxford: EBN Health, 2018.

2   Copson E, Hall P, Board R, et al., eds. Problem solving through precision oncology. Oxford: Clinical Publishing, Oxford, 2017.

3   Board RE, Nathan P, Newsom-Davis T, et al., eds. Problem solving in cancer immunotherapy. Oxford: EBN Health, 2019.

4   Young A, Board RE, Leonard P, et al., eds. Problem solving in acute oncology. 2nd ed. Oxford: EBN Health, 2020.

5   Ring A, Harari D, Kalsi T, et al., eds. Problem solving in older cancer patients. Oxford: Clinical Publishing, 2016.

6   Victoria State Government (2019). Voluntary assisted dying. Available from: www2.health. vic.gov.au/hospitals-and-health-services/patient-care/end-of-life-care/voluntary-assisted-dying (accessed 16 January 2020).

7   Government of Western Australia, Department of Health (2019). Voluntary assisted dying. Available from: ww2.health.wa.gov.au/voluntaryassisteddying (accessed 16 January 2020).

8   New Zealand Herald (2019). Euthanasia bill passes final vote, goes to referendum. Available from: www.nzherald.co.nz/nz/news/article.cfm?c_id=1&objectid=12284896 (accessed 16 January 2020).

Chapter 2: An Oncology Perspective on Choices at the End of Life for Cancer Patients

Ruth E. Board

Introduction

Oncologists are well versed in holding frank and open conversations with patients and their carers about treatment options and prognoses. Often these conversations are difficult, dealing with uncertainty and raw emotions. Towards the end of life, as shared decision making continues, the focus of these conversations shifts subtly to establishing goals for end of life care, hopes for the future, preferred place of care at the end of life and determining what a 'good death) might look like for that individual. For many patients these conversations will ultimately lead to peaceful and dignified dying.

Occasionally patients may request 'a pill) or 'just give me an injection, doc'. Often these are cries for help, borne out of frustration, anger or suffering from an as yet uncontrolled symptom. But sometimes patients have a clear wish for control over the date and timing of their death. Current legislation in the UK rules physician-assisted dying or euthanasia to be illegal. However, this is not the case internationally and a few UK citizens seek the means to end their life abroad. There is a great deal of lobbying and emotive arguments on both sides of the assisted dying debate.

The vast majority of people requesting some form of assisted dying have a cancer diagnosis; therefore, oncologists of all professions need to be able to have open conversations with their patients about choices at the end of life. As assisted dying continues to be debated by the media and parliament, it is crucial that oncologists understand the current legislation both at home and internationally to allow each of us individually to contribute to the debate and be clear about our own personal views on the topic.

Terminology

Box 1.1 in Chapter 1 indicates the definitions used in this text. Euthanasia is the act of intentionally ending a life to relieve suffering: for example, a lethal injection administered by a doctor. This can be voluntary euthanasia, where a person makes a conscious decision to die and asks for help to do so; non-voluntary euthanasia, where a person is unable to give their consent to treatment (for example, if they are unconscious and another person takes the decision on their behalf); or involuntary euthanasia. Intentionally helping another person to kill themselves is known as assisted suicide. Physician-assisted suicide or dying is the term applied when the assistance is given by a physician, for example in prescribing drugs for a patient to self-administer. It should be noted, however, that there is no consensus on these definitions, nor any consistent use of the terms. Assisted dying is felt by some to be a preferable term to use, as opposed to assisted suicide, as it more accurately describes assisted death to reduce unbearable suffering and allows a distinction between suicide or death of those not terminally ill.

Recently, physician-assisted death or medical assistance in dying (MAID) have been more commonly used, usually indicating legally endorsed programmes whereby patients can access

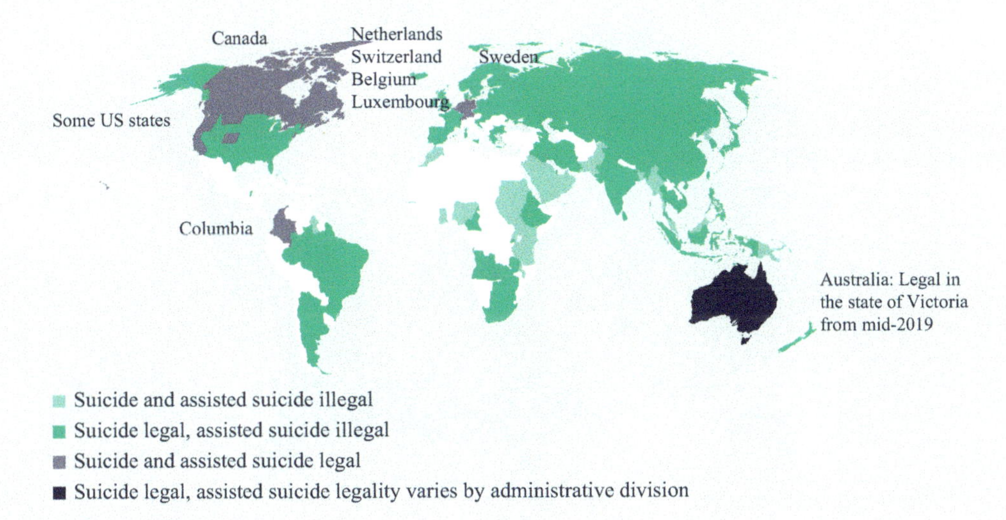

Figure 2.1 Legality of suicide and assisted suicide across the globe (adapted from Borysk5[1]).

voluntary euthanasia or assisted dying. In MAID, a healthcare professional either administers or prescribes medication that intentionally causes the patient's death.

International context

There are worldwide differences in attitudes and legislation on euthanasia and assisted suicide. In many countries, suicide (i.e. the act of taking one's own life) is illegal. In other countries, suicide has been decriminalized, but assisted suicide remains a crime (Figure 2.1).[1] In Canada, Columbia, Luxembourg, the Netherlands, Belgium, Switzerland and parts of Australia, assisted dying has been legalized, although there are differences in the law in terms of access and conditions across those countries. In the USA, assisted dying has been legalized in seven states, namely Oregon, Washington, Washington DC, Vermont, Colorado, Hawaii and California. In Montana, while there is no statute for death with dignity, there is a supreme court ruling recognizing a terminally ill patient's right to die (Figure 2.2).[2] In Canada, the Netherlands, Belgium, Luxembourg and Columbia, both assisted suicide and euthanasia for terminally ill patients are legal. Only in the Netherlands (age >12 years) and Belgium (all ages) is euthanasia by doctors also legal in cases of hopeless and unbearable suffering, even in the absence of a terminal diagnosis. Data show that the most common illness in patients requesting assisted dying is cancer, followed by degenerative neurological conditions. In Oregon, for example, in 2018 the estimated rate of deaths under the Death with Dignity Act was 45.9 per 10,000 total deaths in the state, i.e. 0.45%. Between 1998 and 2017, 77% of patients had a cancer diagnosis and 8% amyotrophic lateral sclerosis.[3]

The debate

Chapter 1 summarizes the history of attempts to change legislation in the UK. The arguments in favour or against assisted dying have been intensely debated in the UK and internationally for many years. The full details of the ethical debate are complex and emotive. In essence, arguments

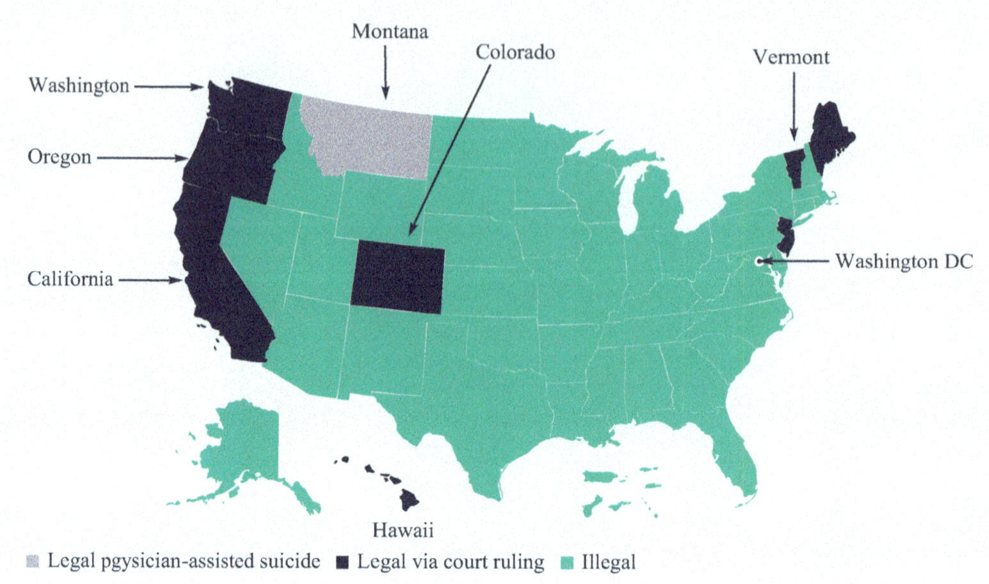

Figure 2.2 US states where physician–assisted suicide is legal (adapted from Terrorist96[2]).

in favour of assisted dying focus on individual autonomy and the right to choose – in this case how, when and where to die. The right to 'die with dignity) without physical or mental suffering is also a central feature of pro-assisted dying arguments. The three most frequently mentioned end of life concerns reported in 2015 by Oregon residents who took advantage of the Death with Dignity Act were: decreasing ability to participate in activities that made life enjoyable (96.2%), loss of autonomy (92.4%) and loss of dignity (78.4%).[3] Those in favour of assisted dying feel that procedural legislation can be put in place to ensure those vulnerable to pressure to accept assisted dying are protected and state that there is increasing public support for some form of assisted dying. The 2017 British Social Attitudes Report[4] demonstrated that the attitude of Britons towards assisted dying had not altered significantly over the last 20 years. Around 80% of those surveyed agreed that the law on assisted dying should definitely or probably be changed to allow voluntary euthanasia where it is carried out by a doctor for a person with an incurable disease. There was less support for other scenarios, e.g. where euthanasia was carried out by a close relative (39%) or where the person was not suffering from a terminal disease (51%) or was completely dependent but not in pain or danger of death (50%).

Conversely, those who do not agree with assisted dying say it is ethically, religiously and/ or morally wrong to kill another person and that legislation cannot fully protect vulnerable members of society. It is argued that assisted dying is the start of a 'slippery slope) leading to non-voluntary or even involuntary euthanasia. They point to the high-quality provision of palliative care, especially in the UK, and the ability of modern medicine to relieve suffering. Some fear that the introduction of euthanasia will reduce the availability of palliative care in the community, because health systems may choose the most cost-effective ways of dealing with dying patients.

The 2015 Quality of Death Index[5] focused on the quality and availability of palliative care to adults and ranked the UK first 'thanks to comprehensive national policies, the extensive integration of palliative care into its National Health Service, and a strong hospice movement'. Palliative care in the UK has been described as being delivered with 'grace and compassion'.[6] It is clear that the debate on assisted dying should not overshadow the need for continued high-quality, easily accessible palliative care.

Opinion of UK oncologists

The Royal College of Physicians (RCP) is a professional body in the UK representing physicians across the globe. Practising medical oncologists in the UK are required to pass the RCP membership (MRCP) exams in order to secure approval for training in medical oncology, the most common training pathway to becoming a UK consultant in medical oncology. In early 2019, the RCP polled its membership of over 35,000 doctors to gather their views on assisted dying.[7] Previously, in a 2014 RCP poll,[8] the majority of respondents did not personally support a change in the law. But there was no majority either way on the question of what the RCP position should be. The 2019 survey was a planned repeat of the 2014 questionnaire.

The RCP defined 'assisted dying) as: 'The supply by a doctor of a lethal dose of drugs to a patient who is terminally ill, meets certain criteria that will be defined by law, and requests those drugs in order that they might be used by the person concerned to end their life.'[7] The RCP stated that the criteria a patient would have to meet would be defined by the law, and, while the RCP could not predict the content of any legislation, it suggested the following:[7] 'Considering past bills, it is likely that two doctors would be required to satisfy themselves that the person making the request:

- was terminally ill (defined as having an incurable and progressive condition as a result of which death is reasonably expected within 6 months);
- had the capacity to make the decision to end their life;
- had the capability to end their life;
- had been fully informed of their palliative care options;
- had a clear and settled intention to end their life, which had been reached voluntarily, on an informed basis and without coercion or duress;
- the legislation would probably also include a conscientious objection clause for all healthcare professionals.'

Importantly the RCP decreed that a supermajority of 60% for a position either supporting or opposing a change in the law would be required. Neutrality would reflect the lack of a simple majority for any particular view.[7]

The following questions were asked of members:

- What should the RCP's position be on whether or not there should be a change in the law to permit assisted dying?
- Do you support a change in the law to permit assisted dying?
- Regardless of your support or opposition to change, if the law was changed to permit assisted dying, would you be prepared to participate actively?
- Is there anything else you want to say about this issue?

The online survey, carried out between 5 February and 1 March 2019, was completed by 6885 respondents from more than 30 medical specialties.[7] The results were as follows:

- What should the RCP's position be on whether or not there should be a change in the law to permit assisted dying?
  - In favour 31.6%
  - Opposed 43.4%
  - Neutral 25.0%
- Do you support a change in the law to permit assisted dying?
  - Yes 40.5%
  - No 49.1%
  - Undecided 10.4%
- Regardless of your support or opposition to change, if the law was changed to permit assisted dying, would you be prepared to participate actively?
  - Yes 24.6%
  - No 55.1%
  - Don't know 20.3%

Comparisons of responses between medical and clinical oncologists show very little variation between the two groups and no significant differences in opinion when compared with the RCP results as a whole (Figure 2.3).

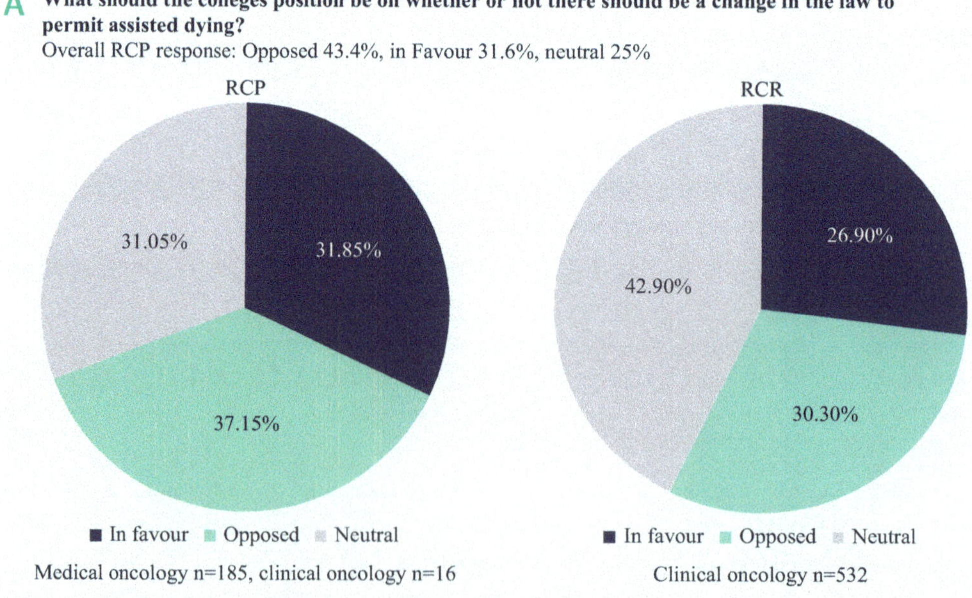

Figure 2.3 (A) What should the colleges) position be on whether or not there should be a change in the law to permit assisted dying? (B) Do you support a change in the law to permit assisted dying? (C) If the law was changed to permit assisted dying, would you be prepared to participate actively?

B **Do you support a change in the law to permit assisted dying?**
Overall RCP response: no 49.1%, yes 40.5%, undecided 10.4%

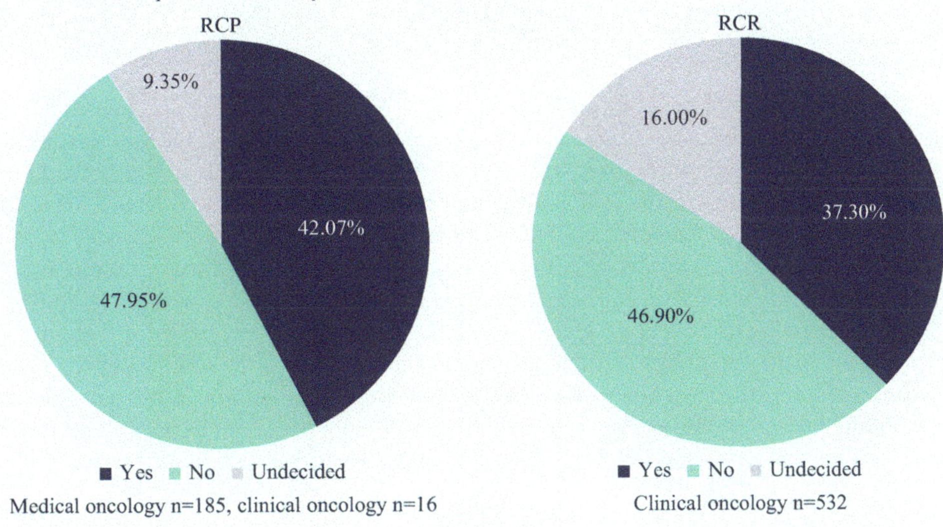

C **If the law was changed to permit assisted dying, would you be prepared to participate actively?**
RCP Overall response: no 55.1%, yes 24.6%, don't know 20.3%

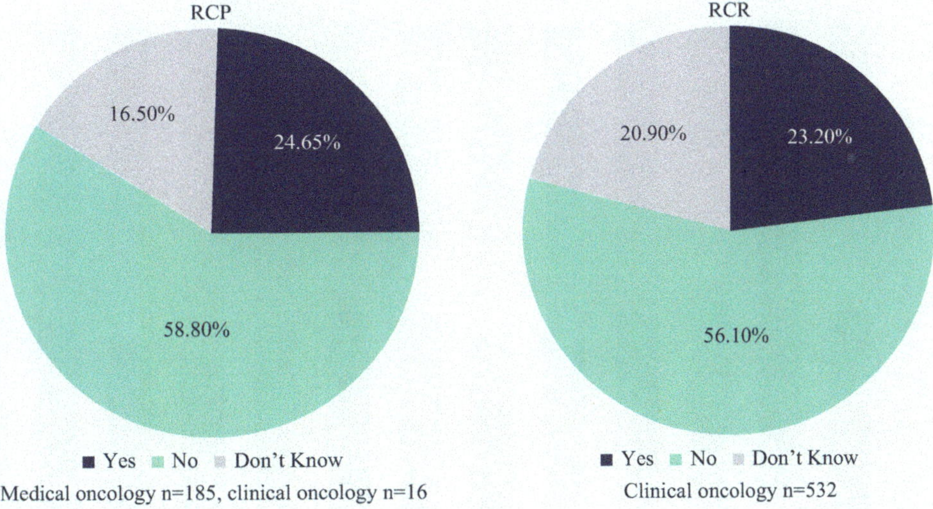

Figure 2.3 (*Continued*)

In response to this poll the RCP dropped its opposition to changing the law on assisted dying and took a neutral stance. RCP president Professor Andrew Goddard said: 'It is clear that there is a range of views on assisted dying in medicine, just as there is in society. We have been open from the start of this process that adopting a neutral position will mean that we can reflect the differing opinions among our membership. Neutral means the RCP neither supports nor opposes a change in the law and we won't be focusing on assisted dying in our work. Instead, we will continue championing high-quality palliative care services.'[9]

In should be noted that while there was no consensus view for the majority of specialties, palliative care physicians voted clearly that the RCP should be opposed to a change in the law on assisted dying (Figure 2.4).[10] The RCP plan to repeat the poll in 2024.

The Royal College of Radiologists (RCR) represents radiologists and clinical oncologists in the UK, where clinical oncologists deliver a substantial proportion of systemic medicine-based treatment for cancer and all radiotherapy. In February 2019, the RCR polled its 1572 UK clinical oncology members and fellows to gain insight into their views on assisted dying.[11] The questions mirrored those of the RCP survey. The results of 532 valid survey responses were presented and the conclusion was that 'the results of this survey show that opinion varies across the faculty of clinical oncology, as would be expected. We do not intend to hold an official faculty of clinical oncology position on assisted dying, but will make these results available publicly.'[11]

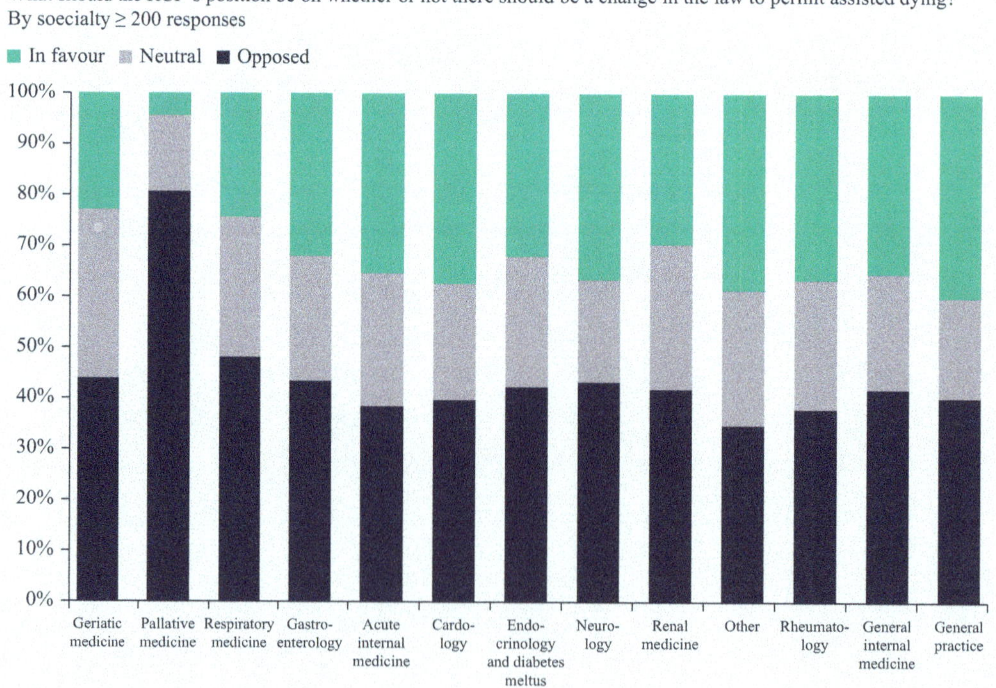

Figure 2.4 RCP survey results by speciality (adapted from Royal College of Physicians[10]).

Conclusion

The patient, public and professional debate on assisted dying continues and is unlikely to disappear. There is a range and depth of personal, professional and religious feeling on both sides of the argument. The changing international landscape and established public opinion in the UK suggest that this debate will continue and that changes in UK law may occur in coming years. It is important that oncologists are equipped with information to help inform patients about their choices at the end of life and to arm themselves with sufficient knowledge to enable them to form their own views on this important topic.

References

1 Borysk5 (2019). Suicide legislation. Available from: https://commons.wikimedia.org/w/index.php?curid=76086863 (accessed 16 April 2019).

2 Terrorist96 (2018). Available from: https://commons.wikimedia.org/w/index.php?curid=39316187 (accessed 16 April 2019).

3 Public Health Division, Center for Health Statistics (2019). Oregon Death with Dignity Act. 2018 data summary. Available from: www.oregon.gov/oha/ph/providerpartnerresources/evaluationresearch/deathwithdignityact/documents/year21.pdf (accessed 19 August 2019).

4 Harding R, The National Centre for Social Research (2017). British social attitudes. 34th ed. Available from: www.bsa.natcen.ac.uk/latest-report/british-social-attitudes-34/key-findings/context.aspx (accessed 19 August 2019).

5 The Economist Intelligence Unit (2015). The 2015 Quality of Death Index. Available from: https://eiuperspectives.economist.com/healthcare/2015-quality-death-index (accessed 19 August 2019).

6 Cannon J. Breaking and mending. London: Profile Books, 2019; 13.

7 Royal College of Physicians (2019). Assisted dying survey. Available from: www.rcplondon.ac.uk/projects/outputs/assisted-dying-survey-2019 (accessed 19 August 2019).

8 Royal College of Physicians (2014). RCP reaffirms position against assisted dying. Available from: www.rcplondon.ac.uk/news/rcp-reaffirms-position-against-assisted-dying (accessed 16 January 2020).

9 Royal College of Physicians (2014). No majority view on assisted dying moves RCP position to neutral. Available from: https://www.rcplondon.ac.uk/news/no-majority-view-assisted-dying-moves-rcp-position-neutral (accessed 16 January 2020).

10 Royal College of Physicians (2019). RCP parliamentary briefing: functioning of the existing law relating to assisted dying. Available from: www.rcplondon.ac.uk/guidelines-policy/rcp-parliamentary-briefing-functioning-existing-law-relating-assisted-dying (accessed 19 August 2019).

11 Royal College of Radiologists (2019). UK clinical oncology members and fellows poll on assisted dying. Available from: www.rcr.ac.uk/posts/uk-clinical-oncology-members-and-fellows-poll-assisted-dying (accessed 19 August 2019).

Chapter 3: How do Permissive Regimes Regulate Assisted Dying?

Penney Lewis

Introduction

A small but growing number of jurisdictions now permit euthanasia and/or assisted suicide. This chapter discusses how the law was changed in those jurisdictions, outlines the regulatory regimes and summarizes the empirical evidence of the practice of euthanasia and assisted suicide (defined in Chapter 1).

How the law was changed to permit assisted dying

The Netherlands

In the Netherlands, euthanasia and assisted suicide were effectively legalized through the use of the defence of necessity in prosecutions of (primarily) doctors. The defence is available when the doctor faced a conflict between his or her duties to preserve life and relieve suffering. The courts held that only doctors could face such a conflict of duties because only doctors had a professional duty to relieve suffering: lay persons (including relatives) and nurses did not. Over some 30 years, the courts developed this duty-based defence of necessity in euthanasia cases, placing conditions on the defence, including: an express and earnest request, unbearable and hopeless suffering, consultation, careful termination of life, record keeping and reporting. These conditions became known as requirements of due care or careful practice. The Dutch legislature eventually codified the parameters of the defence in the Termination of Life on Request and Assisted Suicide (Review Procedures) Act 2001, which lists six due care criteria that must be met in cases of euthanasia and assisted suicide (Box 3.1). The judicially developed necessity defence is still applied to cases involving incompetent persons, particularly neonates.[1,2]

Box 3.1 The Dutch due care criteria.

The due care criteria are set out in section 2(1) of the 2001 Act.
The attending physician must:

a. be satisfied that the patient has made a voluntary and carefully considered request;

b. be satisfied that the patient's suffering was unbearable and that there was no prospect of improvement;

c. have informed the patient about his or her situation and prospects;

d. have come to the conclusion, together with the patient, that there is no reasonable alternative in light of the patient's situation;

e. have consulted at least one other, independent physician, who must have seen the patient and given a written opinion on the due care criteria referred to in a–d above; and

f. have terminated the patient's life or provided assistance with suicide with due medical care and attention.

Belgium

Unlike in the Netherlands, there had been few criminal prosecutions in euthanasia cases prior to its legalization in Belgium, so legal change had to come from outside the judiciary. The 1980s and 1990s witnessed a series of unsuccessful legislative moves to allow euthanasia. After a change of government and intense legislative debate, the law on euthanasia was passed in 2002.[1-3] It allows only doctors to perform euthanasia. Assisted suicide is not explicitly covered, although Belgium's oversight body, the Federal Commission for Euthanasia Control and Evaluation (CFCEE), has accepted cases of assisted suicide as falling under the law.[4] In a recent development, the public prosecution service has taken the position that assisting a suicide is not a criminal offence.[5]

Luxembourg

The law on euthanasia and assisted suicide came into force in Luxembourg in 2009 after a heated political and public debate. The law is closely based on the Belgian law, although it does specifically permit assisted suicide as well as euthanasia.

Switzerland

In Switzerland, it is a criminal offence to assist a suicide only where the assister has a selfish motive. This provision in the penal code has not changed since 1942. When it was originally drafted in 1918, 'The attitudes of the Swiss public were shaped by suicides motivated by honour and romance, which were considered to be valid motives. Motives related to health were not an important concern, and the involvement of a physician was not needed.'[6] Euthanasia is not permitted in Switzerland, although, as in many other European jurisdictions, the separate offence of murder at the victim's request carries a lower minimum sentence than murder.

Oregon and the US states of Washington, Colorado, California, Vermont, Washington DC, Hawaii, New Jersey and Maine (Oregon–model states)

Many US states allow legislation to be enacted if a majority votes for an initiative placed on the ballot following a petition signed by a minimum number of voters. Following two narrowly unsuccessful attempts to permit physician-assisted suicide by ballot initiative in Washington and California, Oregon voters passed the first Death with Dignity Act in 1994 by a majority of 52%. The Act permits the provision of a prescription for lethal medication to be self-administered by the patient. The Act was controversial from the moment the ballot measure was passed, and there were a number of ultimately unsuccessful legal challenges to it.[1] Washington state voters passed an almost identical Act in 2008, as did Colorado voters in 2016. In 2013, 2015 and 2016, respectively, Vermont and California state legislators and District of Columbia council members passed statutes very similar to the Oregon Act, all of which are now in force. The Vermont Act was amended in 2015 to remove certain sunset clauses that would have changed the regulatory framework after 3 years from a regime modelled on Oregon's to a professional practice standard. This would have permitted physician-assisted suicide on the basis of a valid request from a terminally ill patient, without requirements for consultation with a second physician, psychiatric evaluation or waiting periods. The Oregon-model regime will now continue. The Hawaii, New Jersey and Maine legislatures passed Oregon-model Acts in 2018 and 2019.

Colombia

In 1997, the Colombian constitutional court ruled that a physician should not be prosecuted for ending life at the repeated request of a terminally ill patient who was suffering unbearably, because the physician's action was 'justified'. The court called on congress to establish a regulatory regime to vindicate the fundamental right to die with dignity. Although a number of bills were introduced, no progress was made in congress on this issue. In 2014, the constitutional court reviewed the case of a terminally ill patient who had repeatedly and unsuccessfully sought euthanasia. The court ordered the health ministry immediately to issue a directive to healthcare providers requiring them to set up local expert committees to respond to requests for euthanasia. A national expert committee collaborated in the writing of the resulting resolution that came into force in 2015.[7-9]

Canada and Quebec

In 2014, the provincial legislature of Quebec passed an Act respecting end of life care that came into force on 10 December 2015 and legalized euthanasia ('medical aid in dying') for patients at the end of life. In February 2015 in Carter v. Canada, the Supreme Court of Canada struck down the criminal prohibition on assisted suicide found in the federal criminal code, on the grounds that it infringed the rights of competent adult patients with a grievous and irremediable medical condition causing enduring and intolerable suffering who consented to an assisted death.[10] The court granted a 1 year suspension of the declaration of invalidity to give the Canadian parliament the opportunity to craft a regulatory regime. The suspension was subsequently extended by 4 months; during the extension individuals were permitted to access assisted dying by making a court application.[11] Just after the expiry of the extension in June 2016, the Canadian parliament enacted a statute amending the criminal code to permit medical assistance in dying (MAID), which is defined as: '(a) The administering by a medical practitioner or nurse practitioner of a substance to a person, at their request, that causes their death; or (b) the prescribing or providing by a medical practitioner or nurse practitioner of a substance to a person, at their request, so that they may self-administer the substance and in doing so cause their own death.'

Features of assisted dying regimes

This section outlines and compares the features of the main legal regimes permitting assisted dying: those in the Netherlands, Belgium, Luxembourg, Oregon (the model for the eight additional US jurisdictions), Colombia, Quebec and Canada.

The requesting person's condition and experience of suffering

The legal requirements relating to the requesting person's condition and experience of suffering vary widely across these jurisdictions. It is notable that despite this variation, over 70% of all reported cases of euthanasia or physician-assisted suicide involve cancer patients.[12]

In the Netherlands, the 'attending physician ... must have been satisfied that the patient's suffering was unbearable, and that there was no prospect of improvement'. The patient's suffering need not be related to a terminal illness and is not limited to physical suffering such as pain. It can include, for example, the 'fear of future deterioration'.[13] A related due care criterion (Box 3.1) is that there must be 'no reasonable alternative in light of the patient's situation'. In cases where the source of the suffering is a physiological disorder, the patient's reasonable decision to refuse a realistic treatment possibility (whether curative or palliative) that might ease his or her suffering does not stand in the way of a request for euthanasia based on that suffering.

In Belgium, the 'patient [must be] in a medically futile condition of constant and unbearable physical or mental suffering that cannot be alleviated, resulting from a serious and incurable disorder caused by illness or accident'. The patient's suffering need not be limited to physical suffering such as pain. As in the Netherlands, there is no requirement that the patient be suffering from a terminal illness, although additional procedural requirements are imposed if the patient is 'clearly not expected to die in the near future'. Again, there must be 'no reasonable alternative' to euthanasia. However, euthanasia is permissible only if the disorder is incurable; therefore, a patient's reasonable refusal of potentially curative treatment will generally prevent access to euthanasia.[14] The reasonable refusal of a palliative treatment possibility will not have this effect.[15] In recent years, the CFCEE has accepted the possibility that refusal of a potentially curative treatment with particularly serious side effects could be reasonable and would not, therefore, prevent access to euthanasia.[16]

The Netherlands permits assisted suicide in cases where the source of the patient's suffering is a psychiatric rather than a physiological disorder. In such cases, the patient may not reject 'a realistic alternative to relieve the suffering',[17] although 'patients are not obliged to undergo every conceivable form of treatment'.[13] In Belgium, the permissibility of euthanasia in psychiatric cases was initially unclear, but such cases are now accepted by the CFCEE.[15,18]

The Oregon-model states, Luxembourg, Colombia and Quebec all require the diagnosis of a terminal illness, but the Canadian requirement is less clear. In Oregon, the patient must be suffering from a terminal disease, defined as 'an incurable and irreversible disease that has been medically confirmed and will, within reasonable medical judgement, produce death within 6 months'. In Luxembourg, the patient must be in a 'terminal medical situation' and suffering unbearably without prospect of improvement. In Colombia, the patient must be in the terminal phase of an illness or serious pathology, which is progressive, incurable and irreversible, with death predicted in the relatively short term. Similarly, in Quebec, the patient must be at the 'end of life'. The Act requires that the patient 'suffer from a serious and incurable illness, be in an advanced state of irreversible decline in capability, and experience constant and unbearable physical or psychological suffering that cannot be relieved in a manner the patient deems tolerable'. The Canadian Act requires that the patient have a 'grievous and irremediable medical condition', for which there are four criteria: (1) a serious and incurable illness, disease or disability; (2) an advanced state of irreversible decline in capability; (3) the illness, disease or disability or the state of decline must cause the patient enduring physical or psychological suffering that is intolerable to them and that cannot be relieved under conditions that they consider acceptable; and (4) their natural death must have become reasonably foreseeable, taking into account all of their medical circumstances, without a prognosis necessarily having been made as to the specific length of time that they have remaining.

The request

In the Netherlands, the patient must be competent and the request 'voluntary and carefully considered'. Patients aged 16 years and over with capacity may also make an advance written request, which will allow an attending physician to carry out euthanasia in the event of incapacity, provided the due care criteria are met.

In Belgium, the patient must be 'legally competent'. The request must be both 'completely voluntary' and 'not the result of any external pressure'. The doctor must inform the patient about 'his health condition and life expectancy' and 'the possible therapeutic and palliative courses of action and their consequences'. The Act also allows the patient to make an advance request for euthanasia. However, since the triggering condition is irreversible unconsciousness, advance requests will not be applicable to many scenarios of future incompetence, including dementia.

In Oregon, the competence, voluntariness and information requirements are set out in some detail. The patient must have 'the ability to make and communicate healthcare decisions to health-care providers, including communication through persons familiar with the patient's manner of communicating if those persons are available'. Two witnesses must attest that the patient is acting voluntarily and is not being coerced to sign the request. The patient must make an 'informed decision ... that is based on an appreciation of the relevant facts and after being fully informed by the attending physician of: (a) his or her medical diagnosis; (b) his or her prognosis; (c) the potential risks associated with taking the medication to be prescribed; (d) the probable result of taking the medication to be prescribed; (e) the feasible alternatives, including, but not limited to, comfort care, hospice care and pain control'.

In Colombia, the request must be free, informed and unequivocal. In Quebec, the patient must have capacity, be informed and be acting freely. In Canada, the person must be an adult with capacity who has made a voluntary and informed request for MAID.

The requesting person's age

The Dutch law applies both to adults and to patients below the age of majority (18 years). A patient between the ages of 16 and 18 who is 'capable of making a reasonable appraisal of his own interests' may request euthanasia or assisted suicide. A parent or guardian does not have a veto but must be consulted. Patients aged between 12 and 16 must pass the same test of capacity. In addition, the consent of the parent(s) or guardian is required.

In Belgium, euthanasia was originally legal only for patients over the age of 18 and for minors over the age of 15 who had been legally emancipated by a judicial decision. In 2014, the Belgian Act was amended to include minors with the capacity of discernment, although this group of minors must be suffering from a terminal illness in order to access euthanasia. An additional consultation with a child psychiatrist or psychologist is required to verify capacity. The consent of the minor's legal representatives (usually the parents) is also needed.

In Colombia, a 2018 resolution permits euthanasia for children from the age of 6 at their competent, informed and voluntary request. Below the age of 14, parental consent is required. Between the ages of 6 and 12, a psychiatric evaluation is required to ensure the child has attained: (1) exceptional neuro-cognitive and psychological development; and (2) the level of understanding of the concept of death (as irreversible and inexorable) expected of adolescents aged 12 and over.[19]

Children cannot have the required legal capacity to commit suicide in Switzerland, but the position of adolescents is unclear.[20] The Oregon, Luxembourg, Québecois and Canadian laws apply only to patients over the age of 18.

Consultation and referral

All of the regimes require another physician (or nurse practitioner, in Canada) to confirm the fulfilment of the legal requirements. A number of additional functions may be served by a consultation requirement, including quality control, avoidance of idiosyncratic judgements, provision of information to the attending physician, and enablement of effective retrospective scrutiny of actions and decisions.[2]

In the Netherlands, the independent physician must see the patient and give a written opinion on the extent to which the due care criteria are met (Box 3.1). The consultation requirements are more stringent if the patient's suffering is due to a psychiatric disorder.[13] The state-funded programme Support and Consultation on Euthanasia in the Netherlands (SCEN) trains physicians to be consultants and to provide support and advice for doctors treating patients at the end of life. The 'vast majority' of reported euthanasia cases involve an SCEN consultant.[13]

In Belgium, the consulting physician must examine the patient and the medical record and ensure that the suffering requirement has been met. Moreover, if the patient 'is clearly not expected to die in the near future', there is a mandatory additional consultation with either a psychiatrist or a relevant specialist (and a waiting period of at least 1 month). Although a consultation with a palliative care expert is not legally required, many Catholic hospitals in Flanders impose such a palliative filter in addition to the statutory criteria.[21]

In Oregon, the attending physician must refer the patient to 'a consulting physician for medical confirmation of the diagnosis, and for determination that the patient is capable and acting voluntarily'. Further, a counselling referral must be made if either the attending or consulting physician suspects that the patient 'may be suffering from a psychiatric or psychological disorder or depression causing impaired judgment'. Physician-assisted suicide is allowed only if the counsellor determines that the patient is not suffering from such a condition.

In Quebec, the consulting physician was originally required to be independent of both the attending physician and the patient. This was interpreted as meaning that the consulting physician could not be involved in the patient's care. This requirement has now been re-interpreted by the commission on end of life care, so that the consulting physician may have a treating (but not a personal) relationship with the patient.[22]

The person providing assistance

In the Netherlands, the courts originally required that the person providing euthanasia was the patient's treating physician.[2] The current requirement focuses more closely on its purpose: the doctor must know the patient sufficiently well to be able to assess whether the due care criteria are met (Box 3.1).[13]

The Belgian Act requires that the physician have 'several conversations with the patient spread out over a reasonable period of time' in order to be certain of the persistence of the patient's suffering and the enduring character of the request. The Dutch purpose-focused argument (that in order to assess whether the due care criteria are met, the doctor must have some familiarity with the patient) might also be applied in Belgian euthanasia cases. However, the legislative history makes clear that the patient should be able to bypass his or her attending physician if so desired – from which one might infer that there is no requirement for a pre-existing physician–patient relationship.[23]

In Oregon, the attending physician is defined as 'the physician who has primary responsibility for the care of the patient and treatment of the patient's terminal disease'. The evidence suggests that many patients who sought assisted suicide had to ask more than one physician before finding one who was willing to provide a prescription. Over the first 3 years of operation of the Oregon law, only 41% of patients received their prescription from the first physician asked (no further data have been reported).[24] This suggests that in many cases there was no longstanding or pre-existing physician–patient relationship.[25] The median duration of that relationship in Oregon over the first 10 years was 11 weeks. The range was between 0 and 1440 weeks (no further data have been reported).[26] Commentators opposed to the Oregon law have raised the possibility that a patient refused physician-assisted suicide by one physician on the grounds of failing to meet one of the statutory criteria may obtain the prescription from a more accommodating physician.[27]

The laws in Belgium, the Oregon-model states, Quebec and Canada contain conscientious objection provisions. Although there is no such provision in the Dutch law, it is nonetheless clear that 'no doctor has any obligation to accede to a request [for euthanasia], however well founded'.[2] The Royal Dutch Medical Association has reiterated this position, stating that, 'Physicians are not under any obligation to assist in euthanasia. Physicians who have fundamental objections to euthanasia and assisted suicide must be respected in their views.'[28]

Reporting and scrutiny

Termination of life on request and assisted suicide remain criminal offences in the Netherlands. The defences inserted into the penal code by the Act require the doctor to report the case as euthanasia or assisted suicide to the municipal pathologist, who then passes the file to the relevant regional euthanasia review committee. If the committee finds that the doctor did not act in accordance with the due care criteria (Box 3.1), the case is referred to the public prosecution service. Between 1999 and 2018, 111 cases were referred (0.16% of reported cases).[29-35] The first doctor to be prosecuted following these referrals was recently acquitted in a case involving an advance request from a patient with dementia (C 2016–85).[36-39] Lack of, or inadequate, consultation is the most significant reason for referral. Consultation may be considered inadequate if the doctor consulted is insufficiently independent from the attending doctor, or if the consultation takes place too early or too late. Problems with the way in which euthanasia is carried out are the second most significant reason for referral. In recent years, most of these cases involve concerns about the dosage of the coma-inducing sedative administered prior to the muscle relaxant that causes death and the need to ascertain the depth of the patient's coma before administering the muscle relaxant.[29]

Compliance with the Belgian law is monitored by the CFCEE, to which all cases of euthanasia must be reported. Only one case has been reported to the prosecutorial authorities by the CFCEE (in late 2015; 0.008% of reported cases)[40] on the grounds that the patient's suffering was not hopeless and a psychiatrist had not been consulted as is required in cases of suffering stemming from a psychiatric disorder. This case was discontinued in 2019 because it involved physician-assisted suicide that the prosecutorial authorities decided was not a criminal offence.[5] A separate criminal investigation is currently proceeding in a case instigated by the family of a young woman diagnosed with autism, which the CFCEE did not refer to the prosecutorial authorities.[41,42]

In Luxembourg, compliance with the law is monitored by the National Commission for Control and Assessment, which reports biannually. From 2009 to 2016 there were 52 reported cases. No cases have been referred to the prosecutorial or medical authorities.[43]

In Oregon, the physician must report each prescription written under the Act to the Oregon Department of Human Services and report each death resulting from the ingestion of the prescribed medication. A total of 24 physicians were referred by the department to the Board of Medical Examiners between 1998 and 2018 for non-compliance with the provisions of the Oregon Act (1.96% of all reported deaths under the Act). Non-compliance with the Oregon Act identified by the department has been almost exclusively of a clerical nature, the most common items being incomplete or late physician reporting forms or incomplete witness forms (the reason for each referral was provided until 2010).[29-35] In relation to the other Oregon-model states, there is no evidence to suggest that non-compliance with the Washington, California or Vermont Acts is reported to the state medical authorities.

In Colombia, the resolution requires requests for euthanasia to be approved by a special three person multidisciplinary hospital-based committee comprising a specialist in the patient's condition (not the treating physician), a lawyer and a psychiatrist or clinical psychologist. The committee also bears responsibility for ensuring that euthanasia is provided within strict time limits and for accompanying the patient and the family members. A retrospective reporting requirement is also imposed. No reports have been published. Informal data suggest the cumbersome procedure is little used.[44]

Between 10 December 2015 and 31 March 2018, the Quebec commission on end of life care received 1621 reports of MAID, although the number of such deaths was understood to be 1632. By April 2019, the commission had reached decisions on 1498 of these. In 66 cases (4.4%) the commission found that one of the legal requirements had not been met. In 29 of these 66 cases, the consultant physician was not professionally independent of the patient (i.e. was treating the patient). As previously noted, this interpretation of the independent consultation requirement has since been abandoned. Leaving out these cases, the referral rate would be 2.5%. All of the cases were referred to the professional regulatory body.[22,45–47] In Canada, a monitoring system was implemented by regulations in 2018.[48] Interim official data indicate that at least 6749 cases were reported across Canada (including Quebec) between 10 December 2015 and 31 October 2018.[49–51]

Empirical evidence

What is known about the effectiveness of safeguards?

There is an extensive body of empirical evidence relating to the safeguards and criteria outlined above and how they operate in permissive regimes, with the most detail available in the Netherlands, Belgium, Oregon and Switzerland.[15] The evidence from these jurisdictions suggests that the legal criteria that apply to an individual's request for assisted dying are well respected: individuals who receive assisted dying do so on the basis of valid requests; third parties who assist individuals to die do not act unlawfully.[52]

What is known about reporting?

Evidence of the effectiveness of the reporting requirement and the scrutiny of reported cases in the Netherlands, Belgium, Oregon and Switzerland is less consistent. There are no data on the reporting rate in Oregon. The reporting rate within the right to die organizations in Switzerland may be 100%. The reporting rate in the Netherlands rose when regional euthanasia review committees were inserted as a buffer between physicians and the authorities, although the Swiss experience suggests that a buffer may not be needed to encourage reporting if the process leading up to the assistance comprises several layers of administration involving a number of different actors coupled with few legal requirements.[29] The reporting rate is significantly higher (81% in 2015) in the Netherlands than in Belgium (53% in 2007), where legalization occurred more recently.[53–55] The reporting rate has risen over time in the Netherlands; it is not yet known whether this is the case in post-legalization Belgium. 'The major reason for failure to report [a case as euthanasia] is that the physician does not regard the course of action as a life-terminating act.'[56] These unreported cases frequently involve the use of non-typical drugs to cause death (morphine rather than barbiturates and/or muscle relaxants that are typically used in euthanasia cases) and/or a very short life expectancy.[53,57] The number of estimated deaths from euthanasia includes such cases, as it does not rely on doctors' labelling of their own practice. Since almost all cases involving typical euthanasia drugs are reported (97% in 2015; 100% in 2010),[53,56,58,59] this inconsistent labelling now likely accounts for almost all unreported cases. This thesis is supported by anonymous data collected from physicians which indicate that consistently close to 100% of the acts termed by physicians as euthanasia and assisted suicide were reported (99% in 2015; 100% in 2010; 97% in 2005).[53,56]

What is known about vulnerable groups?

In 2007, researchers examined data from the Netherlands and Oregon in order to see whether members of vulnerable groups were more likely to receive MAID (either euthanasia or physician-assisted suicide). They examined the frequency of such assistance in 10 groups of potentially vulnerable patients, defined by gender, age, ethnicity, educational and socioeconomic status, illness and disability. They found 'no evidence of heightened risk ... with the sole exception of people with AIDS'. It should be noted, however, that the lack of Oregon data on pre-existing disabilities weakens the force of this conclusion with respect to disability.[23] The researchers concluded that, 'The available data ... shows that people who died with a physician's assistance were more likely to be members of groups enjoying comparative social, economic, educational, professional and other privileges.'[60]

What is known about the frequency of end of life decisions?

Many of the empirical claims made about the practice of euthanasia and physician-assisted suicide under existing legal regimes misrepresent the data, take it out of context or neglect important comparisons with jurisdictions where these practices are prohibited.[61] Figure 3.1 shows the

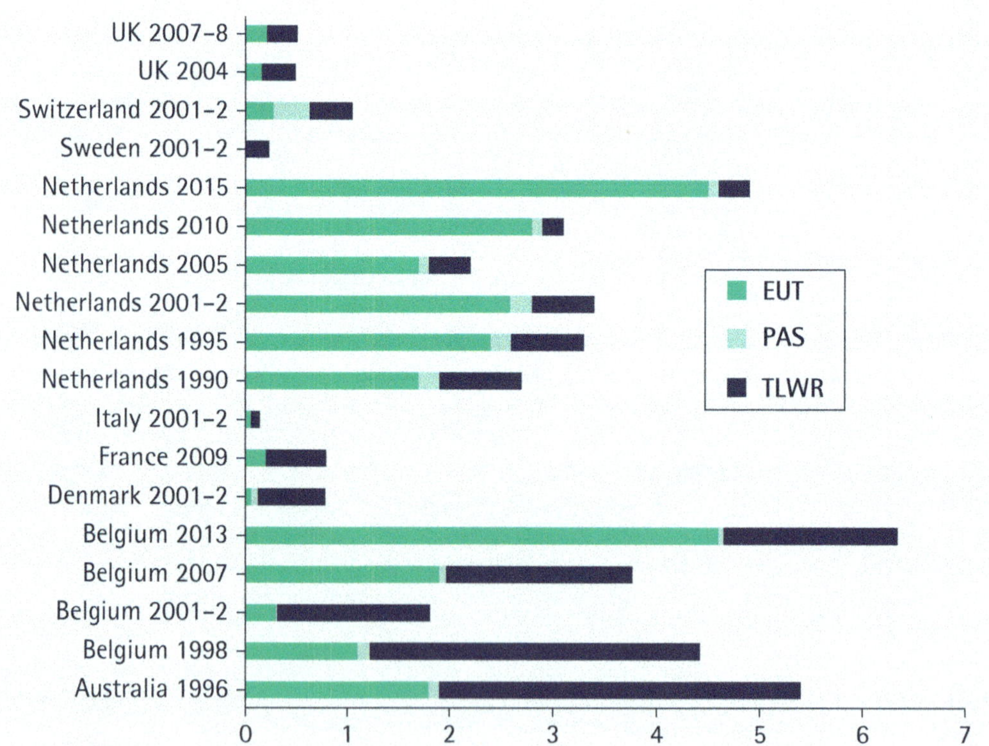

Figure 3.1 Rates of euthanasia (EUT), physician-assisted suicide (PAS) and termination of life without request (TLWR).

percentage of all deaths in specific years that were cases of euthanasia, physician-assisted suicide or termination of life without request. Figure 3.1 combines data from a number of different anonymous prevalence surveys of doctors.[53,55,59,62–70] All surveys were based on one originally designed by Dutch researchers.[70] The relatively broad and overlapping confidence intervals in the surveys suggest that fine comparisons should not be made between countries with the lowest percentages. As indicated, some comparisons are from different years. Although similar, the surveys are not identical. The percentage of deaths in which an end of life decision is made varies across jurisdictions (Figure 3.2).

The evidence does not support the argument that there is a slippery slope between the legalization of euthanasia (termination of life on request) and the termination of life without request.[1,61] The rates of the latter vary. The evidence suggests that termination of life without request takes place in both permissive and non-permissive jurisdictions, with some of the highest rates in non-permissive jurisdictions (e.g. Australia in 1996), although rates of termination of life without request in some permissive jurisdictions are higher than in some non-permissive jurisdictions. Termination of life without request occurs more frequently than euthanasia in all countries that have been surveyed except the Netherlands and Belgium,[71] where rates have decreased since legalization in the permissive jurisdictions of these countries.[1]

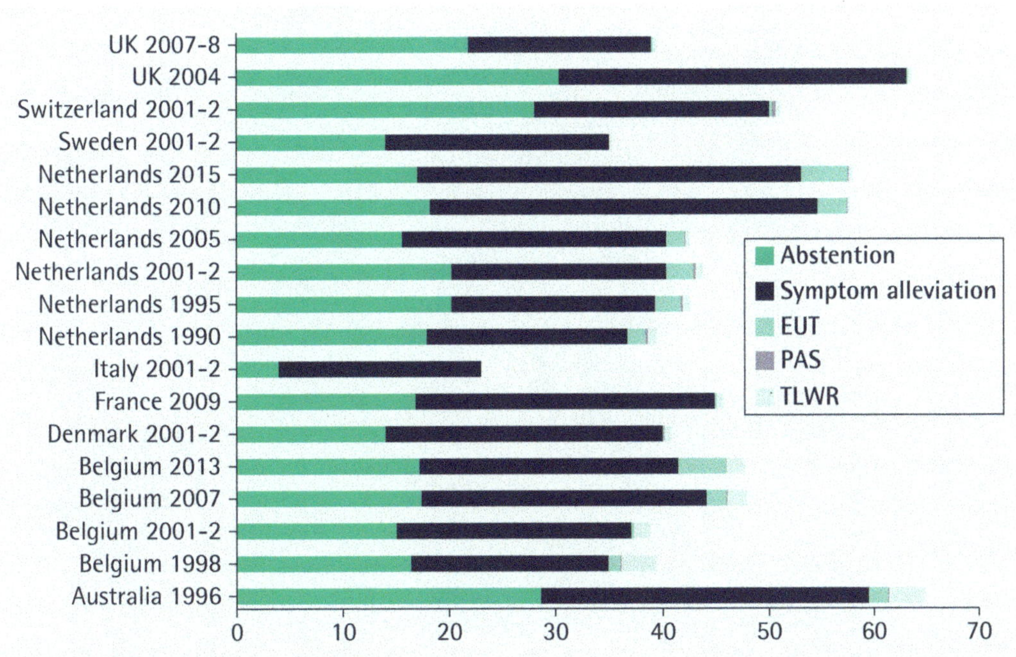

Figure 3.2 Types of end of life decisions in the jurisdictions in which the original Dutch survey was carried out. In addition to euthanasia (EUT), physician-assisted suicide (PAS) and termination of life without request (TLWR), two much larger categories are included: abstention (withdrawing or withholding life-sustaining treatment) and alleviation of symptoms taking into account possible or probable hastening of death. In all countries, EUT, PAS and TLWR are relatively rare.

References

1 Lewis P. Assisted dying and legal change. Oxford: Oxford University Press, 2007.

2 Griffiths J, Weyers H, Adams M. Euthanasia and law in Europe. Oxford: Hart, 2008.

3 Lewis P. Euthanasia in Belgium five years after legalisation. Eur J Health Law 2009; 16: 125–38.

4 Commission fédérale de contrôle et d'évaluation de l'euthanasie. Premier rapport aux chambres legislatives (2002–2003). Brussels: CFCEE, 2004.

5 Arts niet vervolgd voor hulp bij zelfdoding [Doctor not prosecuted for assistance with suicide]. De Standaard 26 April 2019.

6 Hurst SA, Mauron A. Assisted suicide and euthanasia in Switzerland: allowing a role for non-physicians. BMJ 2003; 326: 271–3.

7 Ministerio de Salud y Protección Social, República de Colombia. Resolución 1216 de 2015 por medio de la cual se da cumplimiento a la orden cuarta de la sentencia T-970 de 2014 de la Honorable Corte Constitucional en relación con las directrices para la organización y funcionamiento de los Comités para hacer efectivo el derecho a morir con dignidad. Bogota: Ministerio de Salud y Protección Social, 2015.

8 Ministerio de Salud y Protección Social, República de Colombia. Protocolo para la aplicación del procedimiento de eutanasia en Colombia. Bogota: Ministerio de Salud y Protección Social, 2015.

9 Michalowski S. Legalising active voluntary euthanasia through the courts: some lessons from Colombia. Med Law Rev 2009; 17: 183–218.

10 Carter v. Canada (Attorney General) 2015 SCC 5 (Supreme Court of Canada).

11 Carter v. Canada (Attorney General) 2016 SCC 4 (Supreme Court of Canada).

12 Emanuel EJ, Onwuteaka-Philipsen BD, Urwin JW, Cohen J. Attitudes and practices of euthanasia and physician-assisted suicide in the United States, Canada, and Europe. JAMA 2016; 316: 79–90.

13 Regional Euthanasia Review Committees. Euthanasia code 2018. Review Procedures in Practice. The Netherlands: Regional Euthanasia Review Committees, 2018.

14 Massion J. L'Exception euthanasique en droit Belge. Louvain Méd 2005; 124: 238–45.

15 Lewis P, Black I. The effectiveness of legal safeguards in jurisdictions that allow assisted dying. London: Demos, 2012.

16 Commission fédérale de contrôle et d'évaluation de l'euthanasie. Sixième rapport aux chambres législatives (2012–2013). Brussels: CFCEE, 2014.

17 Office of Public Prosecutions v. Chabot, Nederlandse Jurisprudentie 1994, no. 656 (Supreme Court).

18 Thienpont L, Verhofstadt M, Van Loon T, et al. Euthanasia requests, procedures and outcomes for 100 Belgian patients suffering from psychiatric disorders: a retrospective, descriptive study. BMJ Open 2015; 5: e007454.

19 Ministerio de Salud y Protección Social, República de Colombia. Resolución 825 de 2018 por medio de la cual se reglamenta el procedimiento para hacer efectivo el derecho a morir con dignidad de los niños, niñas y adolescents. Bogota: Ministerio de Salud y Protección Social, 2018.

20 Guillod O, Schmidt A. Assisted suicide under Swiss law. Eur J Health Law 2005; 12: 25–38.

21 Gastmans C, Lemiengre J, van der Wal G, et al. Prevalence and content of written ethics policies on euthanasia in Catholic healthcare institutions in Belgium (Flanders). Health Policy 2006; 76: 169–78.

22 Québec Commission sur les soins de fin de vie. Rapport annuel d'activités 1er juillet 2016–30 juin 2017. Montreal, QC: Québec Commission sur les soins de fin de vie, 2017.

23 Adams M, Nys H. Comparative reflections on the Belgian Euthanasia Act 2002. Med Law Rev 2003; 11: 353–76.

24 Department of Human Services, Oregon Health Division, Center for Disease Prevention and Epidemiology. Oregon's Death with Dignity Act: three years of legalized physician-assisted suicide. Portland, OR: ODHS, 2001.

25 Ganzini L, Nelson HD, Schmidt TA, et al. Physicians' experiences with the Oregon Death with Dignity Act. N Engl J Med 2000; 342: 557–63.

26 Oregon Public Health Division. Tenth annual report on Oregon's Death with Dignity Act: 2010. Portland, OR: Oregon Public Health Division, 2008.

27 Martyn SR, Bourguignon HJ. Now is the moment to reflect: two years of experience with Oregon's physician-assisted suicide law. Elder Law J 2000; 8: 1–56.

28 Royal Dutch Medical Association. KNMG position paper: the role of the physician in the voluntary termination of life. Utrecht: KNMG, 2011.

29 Lewis P, Black I. Reporting and scrutiny of reported cases in four jurisdictions where assisted dying is lawful: a review of the evidence in the Netherlands, Belgium, Oregon and Switzerland. Med Law Int 2013; 13: 221–39.

30 Oregon Public Health Division. Sixteenth annual report on Oregon's Death with Dignity Act: 2013. Portland, OR: Oregon Public Health Division, 2014.

31 Oregon Public Health Division. Seventeenth annual report on Oregon's Death with Dignity Act: 2014. Portland, OR: Oregon Public Health Division, 2015.

32 Oregon Public Health Division. Oregon Death with Dignity Act: 2015. Data summary. Portland, OR: Oregon Public Health Division, 2016.

33 Oregon Public Health Division. Oregon Death with Dignity Act: 2016. Data summary. Portland, OR: Oregon Public Health Division, 2017.

34 Oregon Public Health Division. Oregon Death with Dignity Act: 2017. Data summary. Portland, OR: Oregon Public Health Division, 2018.

35 Oregon Public Health Division. Oregon Death with Dignity Act: 2018. Data summary. Portland, OR: Oregon Public Health Division, 2019.

36 Regional Euthanasia Review Committees. Annual report 2016. The Netherlands: Regional Euthanasia Review Committees, 2017.

37 Miller DG, Dresser R, Kim SYH. Advance euthanasia directives: a controversial case and its ethical implications. J Med Ethics 2019; 45: 84–9.

38 Boffey D. Doctor to face Dutch prosecution for breach of euthanasia law. The Guardian, 9 November 2018.

39 van den Berg S. Dutch doctor acquitted in case of euthanasia of patient with dementia. Reuters, 11 September 2019.

40 Commission fédérale de contrôle et d'évaluation de l'euthanasie. Septième rapport aux chambres législatives (2014–2015). Brussels: CFCEE, 2016.

41 Cheng M. Belgium investigates doctors who euthanized autistic woman. Associated Press, 27 November 2018.

42 Lane C. More trouble for Belgium's system of euthanasia. Washington Post, 29 November 2018.

43 Commission Nationale de Contrôle et d'Évaluation de la loi du 16 mars 2009 sur l'euthanasie et l'assistance au suicide. Quatrième rapport à l'attention de la Chambre des Députés (Années 2015 et 2016). Luxembourg: Commission Nationale de Contrôle et d'Évaluation, 2017.

44 Nolen S. Colombia takes medically assisted death into the morally murky world of terminally ill children. Globe and Mail (Canada), 1 March 2019.

45 Québec Commission sur les soins de fin de vie. Rapport annuel d'activités 10 décembre 2015–30 juin 2016. Montreal, QC: Québec Commission sur les soins de fin de vie, 2016.

46 Québec Commission sur les soins de fin de vie. Rapport annuel d'activités 1er juillet 2017–3 mars 2018. Montreal, QC: Québec Commission sur les soins de fin de vie, 2018.

47 Québec Commission sur les soins de fin de vie. Rapport sur la situation des soins de fin de vie au Québec du 10 décembre 2015 au 31 mars 2018. Montreal, QC: Québec Commission sur les soins de fin de vie, 2019.

48 Regulations for the monitoring of medical assistance in dying, SOR/2018–166, Canada Gazette 2018; 152 (16 part II).

49 Health Canada. Interim update on medical assistance in dying in Canada, June 17 to December 31, 2016. Ottawa, ON: Health Canada, 2017.

50 Health Canada. Second interim report on medical assistance in dying in Canada. Ottawa, ON: Health Canada, 2017.

51 Health Canada. Third interim report on medical assistance in dying in Canada. Ottawa, ON: Health Canada, 2018.

52 Lewis P, Black I. Adherence to the request criterion in jurisdictions where assisted dying is lawful? A review of the criteria and evidence in the Netherlands, Belgium, Oregon, and Switzerland. J Law Med Ethics 2013; 41: 885.

53 Onwuteaka-Philipsen B, Legemaate J, van der Heide A, et al. Derde evaluatie. Wet toetsing levensbeëindiging op verzoek en hulp bij zelfdoding. The Hague: ZonMw, 2017.

54 Smets T, Bilsen J, Cohen J, et al. Reporting of euthanasia in medical practice in Flanders, Belgium: cross sectional analysis of reported and unreported cases. BMJ 2010; 341: c5174.

55 Bilsen J, Cohen J, Chambaere K, et al. Medical end-of-life practices under the euthanasia law in Belgium. N Engl J Med 2009; 361: 1119–21.

56 Onwuteaka-Philipsen B, Gevers JK, van der Heide A, et al. Evaluatie. Wet toetsing levensbeëindiging op verzoek en hulp bij zelfdoding. The Hague: ZonMw, 2007.

57 Buiting HM, van der Heide A, Onwuteaka-Philipsen BD, et al. Physicians' labelling of end-of-life practices: a hypothetical case study. J Med Ethics 2010; 36: 24–9.

58 Rurup ML, Buiting HM, Pasman HR, et al. The reporting rate of euthanasia and physician-assisted suicide: a study of the trends. Med Care 2008; 46: 1198–202.

59 Onwuteaka-Philipsen BD, Brinkman-Stoppelenburg A, Penning C, et al. Trends in end-of-life practices before and after the enactment of the euthanasia law in the Netherlands from 1990 to 2010: a repeated cross-sectional survey. Lancet 2012; 380: 908–15.

60 Battin MP, van der Heide A, Ganzini L, et al. Legal physician-assisted dying in Oregon and the Netherlands: evidence concerning the impact on patients in 'vulnerable' groups. J Med Ethics 2007; 33: 591.

61 Lewis P. The empirical slippery slope from voluntary to non-voluntary euthanasia. J Law Med Ethics 2007; 35: 197–210.

62 Chambaere K, Vander Stichele R, Mortier F, et al. Recent trends in euthanasia and other end-of-life practices in Belgium. N Engl J Med 2015; 372: 1179–81.

63 Deliens L, Mortier F, Bilsen J, et al. End-of-life decisions in medical practice in Flanders, Belgium: a nationwide survey. Lancet 2000; 356: 1806–11.

64 Kuhse H, Singer P, Baume P, et al. End-of-life decisions in Australian medical practice. Med J Aust 1997; 166: 191–6.

65 Pennec S, Monnier A, Pontone S, Aubry R. End-of-life medical decisions in France: a death certificate follow-up survey 5 years after the 2005 Act of Parliament on patients' rights and end of life. BMC Palliat Care 2012; 11: 25.

66 Seale C. End-of-life decisions in the UK involving medical practitioners. Palliat Med 2009; 23: 198–204.

67 Seale C. National survey of end-of-life decisions made by UK medical practitioners. Palliat Med 2006; 20: 3–10.

68 van der Heide A, Deliens L, Faisst K, et al. End-of-life decision-making in six European countries: descriptive study. Lancet 2003; 362: 345–50.

69 van der Heide A, Onwuteaka-Philipsen BD, Rurup ML, et al. End-of-life practices in the Netherlands under the Euthanasia Act. N Engl J Med 2007; 356: 1957–65.

70 van der Maas PJ, van Delden JJ, Pijnenborg L. Euthanasia and other medical decisions concerning the end of life. An investigation performed upon request of the Commission of Inquiry into the Medical Practice Concerning Euthanasia. Health Policy 1992; 21: vi–x, 1–262.

71 Chambaere K, Cohen J. Euthanasia and public health. In: Quah SR, ed. International encyclopedia of public health. Vol. 3. 2nd ed. Oxford: Academic Press, 2017; 46–56.

Chapter 4: Patients, Physicians and Law at the End of Life in England and Wales

Isra Black

Introduction

This contribution has two objectives. The first is descriptive: I provide a brief account of the legal status of a variety of end of life decisions or interventions in England and Wales, including refusal of life-prolonging medical treatment, stopping of eating and drinking (SED), withdrawal or withholding of life-prolonging treatment, euthanasia and assisted suicide. To help set the law in a clinical context, I have included a series of hypothetical cases that a cancer specialist might find challenging if encountered in real life. The second objective is more critical: I consider the legal basis for medicine in England and Wales and attempt to identify the grounds on which physician-assisted death might be argued to be lawful or unlawful compared with other medical interventions.

Four preliminaries: (1) I make no claims as to the applicability of what I say to jurisdictions within the UK other than England and Wales; (2) for brevity, I shall discuss only the law as it applies to individuals aged 18 years and over; (3) again for brevity, I omit discussion of the conferral of lasting powers of attorney; (4) readers should note that by physician-assisted death I mean physician-administered voluntary euthanasia, or physician-assisted suicide. I shall distinguish the former from other kinds of euthanasia in due course.

End of life decisions and interventions and English law

I shall first outline English law as it relates to refusal of life-prolonging treatment, SED, and withdrawal or withholding of life-prolonging treatment. These end of life decisions share common ground, insofar as they involve some combination of a physician offering or not offering medical treatment and a patient consenting to or refusing treatment or being unable to consent or to refuse. I shall then summarize English law on euthanasia and the encouraging or assisting of suicide.

Refusal of life-prolonging treatment

Here our concern is the legal status of the conduct by which a patient declines an intervention offered by a medical professional. A contemporaneous refusal of treatment (or indeed a contemporaneous consent to treatment) is legally valid if the following criteria are met: (1) the physician has informed the patient 'in broad terms of the nature of the procedure';[1] (2) the patient has decision-making capacity, which is governed by the Mental Capacity Act 2005 (MCA 2005), sections 1–3; and (3) the patient's decision is voluntary.[2] If a patient's refusal of treatment lacks validity, it may be lawful to provide treatment, provided that the physician has taken reasonable steps to establish whether the patient lacks capacity, that the physician reasonably believes that the patient lacks capacity, and that the physician reasonably believes that the treatment is in the patient's best interests (MCA 2005, sections 5 and 4).

It is incontrovertible that unless an adult is subject to compulsory treatment under the Mental Health Act 1983, her valid refusal of medical treatment is legally effective. Put another way, the general rule is that overriding a valid refusal of treatment is unlawful, that is, it is a civil wrong (tort) or a crime;[3] the common law (the body of law expounded by judges) takes the *prima facie* inviolability of the person as a fundamental principle.[4] Treatment over a valid refusal is also likely, in the case of physicians engaged in NHS activity, to amount to an unlawful infringement of personal autonomy, which is an aspect of the right to private life protected by article 8 of the European Convention on Human Rights (ECHR) (Human Rights Act 1998 (HRA 1998), sections 6 and 7).[5] Box 4.1 provides a worked example in respect of (contemporaneous) refusal of life-prolonging treatment.

An advance decision to refuse treatment is a decision taken by a person who has decision-making capacity to refuse medical treatment in a future situation in which: (1) she lacks capacity; and (2) a physician wishes to provide the unwanted treatment. The MCA 2005 governs advance decisions to refuse treatment. A key principle of the Act is that 'a person must be assumed to have capacity unless it is established that he lacks capacity) (MCA 2005, section 1(2)). This principle applies as much to advance decisions as it does to contemporaneous refusals of treatment.

A valid and applicable advance decision to refuse treatment has identical legal effect to a valid contemporaneous refusal of treatment (MCA 2005, section 26(1)). Overriding a valid and applicable advance refusal of treatment is unlawful, that is, it amounts to a tort or a crime. In order for an advance decision to refuse treatment to be valid, an individual must not: (1) have withdrawn their decision (MCA 2005, section 25(2)(a); section 24 sets out the modalities for withdrawal (and alteration)); (2) have created a lasting power of attorney *after* the advance decision was made that

---

A 45-year-old woman with breast cancer metastatic to lymph nodes, bone and liver was treated with combination chemotherapy. Initially, she responded well to treatment and obtained a partial remission with good quality of life. This was sustained for 15 months, when she began to develop new symptoms suggestive of recurrence. Reassessment investigations confirmed that she had relapsed at all of the known sites of her disease. Her oncologist offered her a second-line combination chemotherapy, indicating that there was still a good chance that it would reduce the volume of her metastatic disease, improve her symptoms and prolong her life by a few months. They discussed the experience of treatment, the schedule and time commitment required, and the potential for toxicity, including the risks of major toxicity or treatment-related death.

The patient decided to decline second-line chemotherapy and asked that, as has already been considered, she be referred to the palliative care team for symptom control and appropriate end of life care. Her decision was motivated by her wish to spend as much time with her young family as possible. This would be achieved by avoiding hospital trips and the risk of hospitalization.

Is the oncologist obliged to accept a patient's decision to decline a treatment that has a good chance of prolonging life?

The clinician must satisfy herself that the patient's decision is legally valid. She has explained in broad terms the nature of the procedure. The patient is presumed to possess capacity and appears able both to receive the information and process it, and to express her views clearly. There is no evidence that the decision has not been taken voluntarily. As the legal criteria appear to have been met, the patient's decision is legally valid and must be respected. The oncologist and members of the wider multidisciplinary team should support her in her decision.

covers the same subject matter (MCA 2005, section 25(2)(b)). For example, if a person makes an advance decision to refuse cardiopulmonary resuscitation and later makes express provision for the donee of her lasting power of attorney to take all decisions in respect of life-prolonging treatment, the advance decision ceases to be valid; and (3) have done 'anything else *clearly* inconsistent with the advance decision remaining his fixed decision) (MCA 2005, section 25(2)(c)). Whether an individual's behaviour amounts to clear inconsistency requires the exercise of judgement. A good example might be a member of the Jehovah's Witness religion making an advance decision to refuse specific blood products but later renouncing her faith.

A number of factors are relevant to whether an advance decision to refuse treatment is applicable. First, an advance decision is not applicable if an individual is able contemporaneously to consent to or refuse treatment (MCA 2005, section 25(3)). Second, the treatment refused must be the treatment offered and the circumstances in which the treatment is refused must be the circumstances in which the treatment is offered (MCA 2005, section 25(4)(a) and (b)). For example, if a person's advance decision refuses cardiopulmonary resuscitation, but surgery is on offer, the advance decision is not applicable. And if a person's advance decision refuses a blood transfusion in the event that she has dementia, but she has no ongoing neurological disorder and has been involved in a road traffic collision, the advance decision is not applicable. It is important to note that the treatment refused and the circumstances in which the treatment is refused may be specified in lay terms (MCA 2005, section 24(2)). Third, an advance decision is not applicable if 'there are reasonable grounds for believing that circumstances exist that P [the patient] did not anticipate at the time of the advance decision and that would have affected his decision had he anticipated them) (MCA 2005, section 25(4)(c)). Perhaps a classic example of unanticipated circumstances is unforeseen developments in medical treatment (MCA 2005, Code of Practice, paragraph 9.43).[6] Thus, if a person refuses what they expect to be very burdensome treatment, but developments in technology have changed the benefit–burden profile, an advance decision may not be applicable. Finally, an advance decision is not applicable to life-prolonging treatment unless certain conditions are met. The individual must state in her advance decision that she refuses treatment even if her life is at risk (MCA 2005, section 25(5)(a)). And her advance decision must be: (1) in writing; (2) signed by her (or by another person in her presence and acting at her direction); (3) witnessed by a third party – not the same person who signs at the individual's direction; and (4) signed by the witness in the individual's presence.

Stopping of eating and drinking

Although not inherently a medical decision, the pursuit of SED may bring the patient into contact with medical professionals. A patient may decide to refrain from oral ingestion of food and fluids, which is met by an offer to provide clinically assisted nutrition and hydration (CANH) on the part of her physician (or indeed consideration of involuntary feeding by the latter). Or a patient may be in receipt of CANH but wish to refuse it henceforth. Or a patient may wish to receive palliative care, for example, analgesic, antipsychotic or sedative drugs, to improve her dying process.[7] From either of the first two examples the parallel between SED and refusal of treatment emerges: the offer (or contemplation) of medical intervention is met by patient refusal. If an SED decision of this kind is legally valid (the validity criteria are the same as above), it is legally effective in the same way as a refusal of treatment. It is unlawful to feed a patient validly embarking on SED, against her will.[8]

The legal status of support for SED in England and Wales is uncomplicated: it is lawful. The law denies that refusal of life-prolonging treatment ever amounts to suicide.[9] A decision to pursue

> **Box 4.2** Stopping of eating and drinking.
>
> A 67-year-old man was initially diagnosed with locally advanced colon cancer treated by surgery and chemotherapy. He remained well for 15 months, when routine follow-up investigations revealed abnormal liver function tests and imaging revealed liver metastases. He was treated with second-line chemotherapy, followed by the resection of liver metastases. At the end of the procedure he was disease-free on all investigations. A year later the disease returned in the liver and he was treated again with second-line chemotherapy, but surgery was not considered feasible. He experienced considerable toxicity and, after a brief partial regression of his disease, it progressed steadily, producing bulky metastases with associated pain, jaundice and persistent nausea. He became seriously unwell and expressed a wish to have no further active treatment. He discussed the option of further chemotherapy with his oncologist and in a shared decision they agreed that further systemic anticancer treatment was likely to be of very limited benefit.
>
> The patient's symptoms progressed and he decided that he wished to die. He discussed his decision with his family and clinical team. Following the discussion he decided to stop eating and drinking but asked that the clinical team should undertake all measures to keep him as comfortable as possible. The consultant suggested that the patient would be more comfortable if he received intravenous fluids but the patient did not wish to do so.
>
> **Is the consultant permitted to administer intravenous fluids?**
>
> **Are the team permitted to provide symptom control and supportive care through the period during which the patient declines to eat and drink?**
>
> The patient understands the situation and has had the options around systemic anticancer therapy and intravenous hydration explained but declines them. He is presumed to have capacity and there is no evidence to rebut this presumption: he appears able to receive the relevant information, process it and express his views clearly. Similarly, there is no evidence of a lack of voluntariness. The clinical team are therefore not permitted to administer intravenous fluids. They are, however, permitted to provide symptom control until the patient dies or withdraws his decision to refuse nutrition and hydration.

SED in the presence of an offer to provide CANH is a refusal of treatment. In law, such a decision does not constitute suicide. Support for SED cannot amount to suicide assistance, legally speaking. Box 4.2 provides a worked example in respect of SED.

Withholding or withdrawing life-prolonging treatment

Two important common law principles structure the legal regime for withholding or withdrawing life-prolonging treatment. First, a physician owes her patient a common law duty of care 'to take reasonable steps to keep [her] alive) (*R (Burke) v General Medical Council*, paragraph 32).[10] Second, a court will not order a doctor to treat contrary to her clinical judgement.[10,11] It is helpful to treat separately patients who possess decision-making capacity and patients for whom capacity is absent, either on a temporary or a permanent basis, when examining the application of these principles.

In respect of patients who possess decision-making capacity, a valid refusal of treatment extinguishes the physician's duty of care in respect of the treatment offered; the physician has no duty to provide said treatment. Indeed, as noted above, it would be unlawful at common law to force treatment. In situations in which a patient possesses decision-making capacity and wishes to receive life-prolonging treatment, the courts have ruled that a failure to take reasonable steps to keep the patient alive would leave a physician open to a charge of murder (*R (Burke) v General Medical Council*, paragraph 34).[10] This may appear to sit uneasily with the principle that a court will not order a physician to treat contrary to her clinical judgement. In fact, it is perfectly consistent. The civil courts will not order a physician to provide treatment. But she may be open to criminal prosecution should she refuse to treat a patient with capacity who wishes to be kept alive. Box 4.3 provides a worked example in respect of withdrawal of treatment in circumstances in which an individual has decision-making capacity.

Concerning patients who lack decision-making capacity, the physician's legal duty to take reasonable steps to keep her patient alive is conditioned by the requirement that treatment for an individual who lacks capacity will only be lawful if it is in a patient's best interests (MCA 2005, sections 5 and 4). When considering best interests, the legal question is 'whether it is in the patient's best interests to give the treatment, rather than … whether it is in his best interests to withhold or withdraw it) (*Aintree University Hospitals NHS Foundation Trust v James*, paragraph 22).[12] This is because the law's commitment to inviolability of the person applies as much to individuals who lack capacity as it does to individuals who possess capacity;[13] that is, there will be circumstances in which withdrawal or withholding of treatment is required because its provision is not in the patient's best interests. For example, treatment may not be in an individual's best interests when it involves an 'extreme degree of pain, discomfort or indignity) (*R (Burke) v General Medical Council*, paragraph 33),[10] or when an individual is in a permanent or minimally conscious state.[9,14] In all cases, physicians tasked with ascertaining the best interests of an individual who lacks capacity must 'look at his welfare in the widest sense, not just medical but social and psychological … [they

---

Box 4.3 **Withholding or withdrawing life-prolonging treatment.**

A 69-year-old woman was diagnosed with stage 4 non-Hodgkin lymphoma and treated initially with combination chemotherapy. She entered a complete remission. This was maintained for 3 years, when her disease relapsed with rapidly progressive lymphadenopathy and hepatosplenomegaly. Her haemato-oncologist recommended second-line combination chemotherapy and discussed the procedure with her carefully, including the risks of toxicity and the schedule of hospital visits involved. The patient was the principal carer for her husband who was suffering from advanced dementia. She felt that if she spent time away from him it would cause him great distress. She declined chemotherapy and asked for an active programme of symptom control and support at home.

The haemato-oncologist was greatly concerned by the patient's refusal of a treatment that he considered would bring her considerable benefit. He felt that he would be failing in his duty of care were he not to deliver the chemotherapy. He sought legal advice from his NHS trust.

What is the legal advice?

The legal advice states in the event that the patient fulfils the criteria for a valid refusal of treatment. Her refusal of treatment relieves the physician of his duty of care to prolong her life by providing chemotherapy. He may continue to provide her with general medical care and involve other professionals as necessary to ensure symptom control and end of life care when appropriate.

must] put themselves in the place of the individual patient and ask what his attitude to the treatment was or would be likely to be) (*Aintree University Hospitals NHS Foundation Trust v James*, paragraph 39).[12]

Approaching best interests from a patient-centred and welfare-driven perspective may mean that physicians become legally required to discontinue treatment, contrary to their clinical judgement. It does not entail, however, that physicians are required to treat patients when treatment runs contrary to their clinical judgement (*R (Burke) v General Medical Council*, paragraph 31),[10] subject to the requirement that the exercise of professional discretion is reasonable (*Aintree University Hospitals NHS Foundation Trust v James*, paragraph 22).[12,15] Again, no court will order a physician to provide treatment contrary to her clinical judgement. Moreover, no court will hold that an intervention is in a patient's best interests if there is no physician who is 'ready, willing and able) to provide treatment; speculative applications to the court for determination of best interests will be struck out for abuse of process.[16]

Euthanasia

Euthanasia involves a person (D) deliberately causing the death of another (P), for P's own good. A classic example of euthanasia relevant to our discussion involves a physician deliberately injecting her patient with lethal medication because it is *better* or *best* for the latter. We may further describe euthanasia as voluntary, non-voluntary or involuntary. Voluntary euthanasia involves D causing P's death, for P's own good, when P has consented to D's conduct. Non-voluntary euthanasia involves D causing P's death, for P's own good, when P lacks capacity to consent to D's conduct. Involuntary euthanasia involves D causing P's death, for P's own good, when P has refused D's conduct (that is, death is imposed against P's will). Only voluntary euthanasia performed by a physician falls within the rubric of physician-assisted death.

All forms of euthanasia are illegal (that is, constitute murder) in English law (*Airedale NHS Trust v Bland*, page 865).[9] The offence is made out regardless of whether the person who dies consented to the conduct causing her death, or that death was better or best for her; that is, consent is no defence to murder and there is no distinction between euthanasia and less beneficent killing. Box 4.4 provides a worked example in respect of voluntary euthanasia.

An 89-year-old man had advanced unresectable recurrent rectal cancer that was producing obstruction at the rectosigmoid junction. He had delayed attending for medical care and the complications progressed to include a perforation producing intractable peritonitis and persistent difficulty to control pain. He was treated with antibiotics and intravenous hydration, but a surgical consultant confirmed that no operation could prevent the leakage of bowel contents into the peritoneal cavity.

The patient understood the situation and considered all the procedures that were options for him. He was particularly distressed by the loss of dignity experienced in association with his extensive intra-abdominal complications. He asked a member of the clinical team if it was possible to have euthanasia.

Are the clinical team permitted to provide euthanasia?

Euthanasia is unlawful in all jurisdictions within the UK. The clinical team are not permitted to provide euthanasia.

Assisted suicide

Suicide ceased to be a crime upon the enactment of the Suicide Act 1961, section 1. However, the Suicide Act 1961, section 2(1), makes encouraging or assisting suicide a crime. Under the Act, '(«D«) commits an offence if (a) D does an act capable of encouraging or assisting the suicide or attempted suicide of another person, and (b) D's act was intended to encourage or assist suicide or an attempt at suicide'. An example of physician-assisted suicide that would fall within the scope of the offence is the prescription by a physician of a lethal dose of barbiturates to her patient, which the latter self-administers.

The consent of the Director of Public Prosecutions (DPP) is required for any prosecution for encouraging or assisting suicide (Suicide Act 1961, section 2(4)). In exercising the discretion, the DPP applies the two-stage test contained in the Code for Crown Prosecutors,[17] supplemented by an offence-specific policy on encouraging or assisting suicide.[18] The first stage of the test requires prosecutors to consider whether 'there is sufficient evidence to provide a realistic prospect of conviction) (Code for Crown Prosecutors, paragraph 4.6).[17] If this stage is passed (a case cannot otherwise proceed), the prosecutor must consider whether criminal proceedings are in the public interest. Here, the policy on encouraging or assisting suicide becomes relevant. The policy enumerates a number of factors that tend in favour and that tend against prosecution. These factors principally concern the determination of whether an individual's decision to perform suicide is autonomous.[19] For example, factor 3 tending in favour of prosecution reads, 'the victim had not reached a voluntary, clear, settled and informed decision', while factor 5 tending against prosecution reads, 'the actions of the suspect may be characterized as reluctant encouragement or assistance in the face of a determined wish on the part of the victim'.[18]

In respect of physician-assisted suicide, health professional status is a factor that tends in favour of prosecution, albeit not in and of itself. Factor 14 of the policy on encouraging or assisting suicide states that prosecution is more likely if 'the suspect was acting in his or her capacity as a medical doctor, nurse, other healthcare professional, a professional carer [whether for payment or not] ... and the victim was in his or her care'.[18]

Factor 14 includes the following clarificatory footnote: 'the words "and the victim was in his or her care" qualify all of the preceding parts of this paragraph ... This factor does not apply merely because someone was acting in a capacity described within it: it applies only where there was, in addition, a relationship of care between the suspect and the victims [sic] such that it will be necessary to consider whether the suspect may have exerted some influence on the victim.'[18]

Again, we can see that the issue is whether the individual's suicide is autonomous, or whether the professional's influence is such that there would be worries that the deceased's decision was not voluntary; that is, it is not professional status alone that is a factor that tends in favour of prosecution for the Suicide Act 1961, section 2, offence. Rather, it is professional status in conjunction with a relationship of care. However, to the extent that it is potentially difficult to conceive of circumstances in which a physician provides *medical* suicide assistance in the absence of a relationship of care, it may be difficult to avoid investigation into the degree of influence exerted on the deceased. For example, it seems plausible that if a physician prescribes medication knowing that an individual will stockpile it and attempt suicide, she does so within the context of a duty of care owed to the patient.

Before moving on, we should note the successive stream of litigation seeking to effect permissive legal change on assisted death since the entry into force of the HRA 1998 in October 2000. The offence-specific prosecutorial policy on encouraging and assisting suicide owes its existence to the decision in *R (Purdy) v DPP*,[20] in which the House of Lords held that the Code for Crown

Prosecutors failed to provide sufficient clarity as to the DPP's exercise of discretion to prosecute under the Suicide Act 1961, section 2(4). As such, the interference caused by the prohibition on encouraging or assisting suicide with the right to respect for private life protected by article 8 of the ECHR was not 'in accordance with the law'.[20] The decision in *R (Purdy) v DPP* was made possible by the ruling of the ECHR in *Pretty v United Kingdom* that the right to decide how and when to die is an aspect of the right to private life protected by article 8 of the ECHR.[21] Unsuccessful challenges to the law on assisted death have followed.[22–24] More litigation on the issue of whether the criminal prohibition on assisted death is compatible with article 8 of the ECHR is highly likely. In parallel to activity in the courts, the campaign organization Dignity in Dying is spearheading ongoing attempts to legalize a version of the Oregon model for physician-assisted suicide through Parliament (see, for example, the Assisted Dying (No. 2) Bill 2015–16 and the Assisted Dying Bill [HL] 2015–16). Box 4.5 provides a worked example in respect of suicide assistance.

Box 4.5 Suicide assistance.

A 75-year-old man had locally advanced prostate cancer treated by radiotherapy and hormone therapy. He obtained a useful remission of his disease with good quality of life. Unfortunately, 18 months later the disease in the pelvis progressed, resulting in extensive bone metastases producing painful fractures. He was treated with intravenous chemotherapy and targeted therapy, with very little benefit. He received radiotherapy to painful bone lesions that reduced his pain considerably for several months.

During the period of reasonable symptom control, the patient decided in view of his age, his frailty and his social situation that he wished to travel to a Switzerland where he could lawfully perform suicide with the assistance of an organization that provides this service.

He asks his clinical team if they would prepare a report documenting his case and explaining his clinical status that could be provided to the organization in the jurisdiction in which assisted suicide is lawful. He had no family or friends and he asked the clinical team if they would assist him in booking ambulance-assisted air travel to the other country to receive assistance to die.

Are the clinical team permitted to prepare a report for him to help him make his arrangements?

The clinical team are entitled to refuse to write a medical report for the patient because of the risk of exposure to criminal liability. The provision of a report is an act capable of encouraging or assisting suicide or attempted suicide. If the report is intended to encourage or assist suicide, the issue of criminal liability will arise. Writing a medical report for the patient also runs the risk of professional regulatory fitness-to-practise proceedings.[25,26]

A patient may request a copy of his medical records, which the clinical team are under a legal obligation to provide. Paragraph 22 of the General Medical Council (GMC) guidance states that compliance with a data subject access request will 'not normally give rise to a question of impaired fitness to practise'.[25]

Some actions related to a person's decision to, or ability to, commit suicide are lawful, or will be too distant from the encouragement or assistance to raise a question about a doctor's fitness to practise. These include, but are not limited to, 'providing access to a patient's records where a subject access request has been made in accordance with the terms of the (Data Protection Act 2018, section 45)'.[25]

The GMC position can be explained by 'legal advice to the effect that a doctor's compliance with a subject access request even if they knew the reason for that request [was to seek assisted suicide] would be too far removed from the act of suicide to constitute encouragement or assistance'.[27] This provides insight into the legality of complying with a request for medical records that a patient intends to use for the purposes of suicide assistance. Such conduct is unlikely to constitute an act capable of encouraging or assisting suicide; it falls outside the bounds of the Suicide Act 1961, section 2, offence.

Are they permitted to help him book his flight with appropriate clinical and ambulance support?

This conduct falls within the scope of the offence of encouraging or assisting suicide. The first stage of the two-stage test would likely be satisfied; that is, there would be sufficient evidence (such as correspondence regarding transit arrangements) to provide a realistic prospect of a conviction. In respect of the second, public interest, stage, the patient's apparently autonomous decision to seek suicide assistance abroad would be a factor tending against prosecution. However, the pre-existing duty of care between the clinical team and the patient would constitute a factor tending in favour of prosecution. Even if it were ultimately concluded that prosecution was not in the public interest, the mere fact of the duty of care will likely result in a police investigation into the conduct of the clinical team.

What's so (legally) special about physician–assisted death?

Physician-assisted death, that is, physician-administered voluntary euthanasia and physician-assisted suicide, is unlawful in England and Wales. In this section, I wish to interrogate the idea that, legally speaking, physician-assisted death is special compared with other medical interventions. I consider, through discussion of the *medical exception* (the legal doctrine that 'takes most medical treatment outside ... criminal law regulation'[28]) what it is that might make physician-assisted death legally exceptional.

I argue that in terms of patient benefit, the reasons a physician might provide assistance to die may be the same as the reasons she might offer other medical interventions. On this ground, physician-assisted death is not legally special. However, it is possible that physician-assisted death may be legally differentiated from other medical interventions on public interest grounds. It is these latter arguments that require careful specification and evaluation. If it is plausible that physician-assisted death falls within the medical exception, we have reason to think that it ought to be lawful.

I should stress that what follows is a legal argument, as opposed to a moral argument. Of course, the separation between law and morality is not always neat, and the discussion touches on factors that might be thought relevant to the moral permissibility of physician-assisted death and assisted death more broadly.

What is the medical exception? It is important to recognize that the criminal law is of universal application and is *prima facie* applicable to medical conduct. Medical interventions that involve bodily interference or conduct that causes injury would be crimes, often serious crimes, were it not for legal rules that exempt medicine from the criminal law (*R v Brown*, page 266).[29]

A general principle of the criminal law is that consent alone makes bodily interference involving touching but amounting to less than actual bodily harm lawful.[29] A physician does not commit a crime in touching her patient during a medical examination and treatment, because the latter has waived her inviolability through consent. If, during the course of medical intervention, a physician injures her patient (causes actual bodily harm or greater), consent alone does not provide a defence; the conduct is *prima facie* criminal, but the medical exception may render it lawful. Here, injury refers to any event that interferes with the health of the patient, even if she will be better off overall if treatment is successful. For example, injury may include tissue damage from injections or catheterization, wounds from surgical incision, or the main and side effects of chemotherapy. The medical exception makes these instances of injury-causing conduct lawful because there is a public interest in the practice of medicine.

Penney Lewis observes three categories of public interest reasons that may explain why a particular intervention falls within the medical exception: (1) patient-focused – the intervention is better for patients (by which is meant any potential class of patients); (2) public-focused – the intervention is better for the community (which might include its being better for patients), for example, tissue and organ donation and non-therapeutic research; (3) professionally focused – the intervention accords with accepted medical practice.[28]

I shall focus on the patient-focused and public-focused reasons. While professionally focused reasons may explain why an intervention falls within the medical exception, I am dubious as to whether appeals to accepted medical practice can, in and of themselves, justify or determine its legality. Any compelling appeal to why it is professionally appropriate to offer an intervention must surely rely on patient- or public-focused reasoning. Importantly for my purposes, physicians have no monopoly over what counts as patient or community benefit. We can employ these concepts to evaluate whether physician-assisted death ought to fall within the medical exception, and for what reason.

In respect of patient benefit, the argument is that it is in the public interest for medical interventions that are better for patients to stand outside the criminal law (within the medical exception). Typically, the analysis of whether a procedure is better for patients involves a *welfare-level comparison*. Would an individual be better off in terms of her well-being were she to have the intervention compared with not having it? Implicit in this analysis is the patient's continued existence regardless of whether she receives treatment. For example, the choice whether to have knee surgery may involve the option of surgery with the promise of greater mobility, and the option of reduced mobility without surgery. In the ordinary run of things, this decision involves choosing between states of affairs in which the patient is alive.

It is intuitive that assisted death could be better for some individuals: for example, those who suffer and wish to die, whose suffering is grave and for whom death would be a proportionate response.[30] However, the analysis of whether physician-assisted death falls within the medical exception cannot appeal to welfare-level comparisons; that is, we cannot establish its betterness for patients by thinking comparatively about well-being in the usual way. This is because if an individual receives assistance to die, she will cease to exist; whereas, if she does not, she will, at least for a time, continue to exist. A welfare-level comparison in such circumstances is impossible: it involves comparing existence and non-existence, something and nothing. In order for physician-assisted death to fall within the medical exception, it is necessary to describe how it could be better for patients in a *non-welfare-level comparison* sense. This may be philosophically challenging.[31]

Importantly, however, resort to non-welfare-level comparisons does not make physician-assisted death legally special. There are interventions whose situation within the medical exception can only be explained by appeal to non-welfare-level comparisons. This is the case for life-prolonging interventions as a class. For example, when considering whether surgical treatment for mortal (gunshot, knife, etc.) wounds is better for patients, we must compare the option of surgery and (it is hoped) living, with the option of not having surgery and dying: we must compare the comparative value of existence and non-existence. Ordinarily, it is lawful to treat mortal wounds because it is better for patients, but the analysis of why it is better to have life-prolonging treatment does not involve a comparison of welfare levels of a person who will exist regardless of whether they have treatment. In sum, the fact that physician-assisted death requires a non-welfare-level analysis of patient benefit cannot exclude it from falling within the medical exception; that is, if assisted death is better for patients, it may be lawful for the same reason that other medical interventions are lawful.

According to the public-focused justification, interventions that are better for the community are in the public interest and fall within the medical exception. As noted above, this includes interventions whose benefit to the individual who undergoes the procedure is questionable, such as tissue and organ donation and non-therapeutic research. In addition, it is plausible that it is in the interest of the community that individuals receive interventions that are better for them. As such, the public-focused justification for the medical exception might be thought to include the patient-focused justification. There is, I would argue, an important qualification to this claim: an intervention that is better for patients cannot be worse for the community in terms of its impact on its members) rights or interests. For example, in the North Carolina case of *State v Bass*, it was (arguably) better for the patient to have his hand anaesthetized (by a doctor) prior to amputation of four digits (by someone else) in order to commit insurance fraud, but it is clearly worse for the community to facilitate such crimes.[32] This constraint on the compatibility of patient- and public-focused justifications for the medical exception potentially points to a basis for legal differentiation of physician-assisted death from other medical interventions.

While physician-assisted death may be better for patients, it might be thought to exert harmful effects on the community. The challenge for proponents of the legalization of assisted death who wish to bring physician-assisted death within the medical exception is to show that it would not be the case, and the challenge for opponents of legalization is to show that it would be the case.

The English courts have identified three principal arguments against the legalization of assisted death, none of which are settled. First, it might be thought that the legal permissibility of assisted death exposes certain populations, for example, individuals who might be exposed to pressure to seek assistance to die or socialized into thinking that their lives are not worth living, to the risk of harm, and that risk justifies disregarding the benefits of legalization for others.[22,33] Second, it might be thought that the legalization of physician-assisted death would undermine trust between patients and doctors.[23] Third, it might be thought that legalization of physician-assisted death expresses or communicates the view that human life under certain conditions may not be worth living, and that it is wrong for the law to express this sentiment (*R (Nicklinson and Another) v Ministry of Justice*, paragraphs 91 and 185)).[22]

I do not intend (and I lack the space) to resolve these arguments here. What is important to note is that none seem to be pressing issues in respect of currently lawful medical interventions – though the second occasionally comes up in various forms in respect of organ transplantation.[34] On the one hand, it is possible that physician-assisted death is legally special because of one or more of these grounds. This would mean that physician-assisted death would be incompatible with the public-focused justification for the medical exception and as such ought not to be lawful for the same reason that other medical interventions are lawful. On the other hand, if none of these arguments have merit, all things considered, physician-assisted death would not be legally special and there we would have a compelling reason to think that it ought to be lawful and treated like any other (lawful) medical procedure. It is necessary carefully to specify and to evaluate each of the worse-for-the-community-based objections to the legalization of physician-assisted death in order to establish the truth.

Conclusion

This contribution had two aims. First, I sought to provide an overview of the legal status of a variety of end of life decisions or interventions in England and Wales. Refusal of life-prolonging medical treatment, SED, and withdrawal or withholding of life-prolonging treatment are all lawful in this jurisdiction. Euthanasia and assisted suicide are both unlawful. Second, I explained what makes medicine lawful in England and Wales. I applied analysis of the medical exception – the legal doctrine that exempts procedures involving injury to the patient from the criminal law – to physician-assisted death. I argued that physician-assisted death may be better for patients in the same way as other medical interventions may be better for patients. I also outlined three potential arguments that physician-assisted death might be worse for the community and thus not able to fall within the medical exception: the risk of harm to others; trust in the medical profession; and the purported expression in law that some lives are not worth living. These arguments involve complex empirical or normative matters, but it behoves us to attempt to resolve them and establish whether assisted death has a place in medicine.

Acknowledgements

I would like to express my gratitude to Peter Selby, for his editorial support and for drafting the worked examples, and to Penney Lewis, for her editorial comments that improved the argument and its clarity. I would also like to thank Lisa Forsberg, who read drafts of this contribution. The responsibility for errors is mine only.

References

1   *Chatterton v Gerson* [1981] QB 432.

2   *Re T (Adult: Refusal of Treatment)* [1993] Fam 95.

3   *Ms B v an NHS Hospital Trust* [2002] EWHC 429.

4   *Collins v Wilcock* [1984] 1 WLR 1172.

5   Black I. Refusing life-prolonging medical treatment and the ECHR. Oxf J Leg Stud 2018; 38: 299–327.

6   Department for Constitutional Affairs. Mental Capacity Act 2005. Code of Practice. London: TSO, 2007.

7   Wax JW, An AW, Kosier N, Quill TE. Voluntary stopping eating and drinking. J Am Geriatr Soc 2018; 66: 441–5.

8   Huxtable R. Whatever you want? Beyond the patient in medical law. Health Care Anal 2008; 16: 288–301.

9   *Airedale NHS Trust v Bland* [1993] 1 AC 789.

10 *R (oao Burke) v General Medical Council* [2005] EWCA Civ 1003.

11 Re J (A Minor) (Wardship: Medical Treatment) [1991] Fam 33.

12 *Aintree University Hospitals NHS Foundation Trust v James* [2013] UKSC 67.

13 *Wye Valley NHS Trust v B* [2015] EWCOP 60.

14 *Briggs v Briggs* [2016] EWCOP 53.

15 *Bolam v Friern Hospital Management Committee* [1957] 1 WLR 582.

16 *AVS v an NHS Foundation Trust* [2011] EWCA Civ 7.

17 Crown Prosecution Service. The Code for Crown Prosecutors. 8th ed. London: Crown Prosecution Service, 2018.

18 Crown Prosecution Service (2014). Policy for prosecutors in respect of cases of encouraging or assisting suicide. Issued by the Director of Public Prosecutions. February 2010 (updated October 2014). London: CPS, 2014.

19 Montgomery J. Guarding the gates of St Peter: life, death and law making. Leg Stud 2011; 31: 644–66.

20 *R (oao Purdy) v DPP* [2009] UKHL 45.

21 *R (oao Pretty) v DPP* [2001] UKHL 61.

22 *R (oao Nicklinson and Another) v Ministry of Justice; R (oao AM) v DPP* [2014] UKSC 38.

23 *R (oao Conway) v Secretary of State for Justice* [2018] EWCA Civ 1431.

24 *R (oao Newby) v Secretary of State for Justice* [2019] EWHC 3118.

25 General Medical Council (2013). Guidance for the investigation committee and case examiners when considering allegations about a doctor's involvement in encouraging or assisting suicide. Available from: www.gmc-uk.org/-/media/documents/DC4317_Guidance_for_FTP_decision_makers_on_assisting_suicide_51026940.pdf (accessed 16 January 2020).

26 General Medical Council (2013). Patients seeking advice or information about assistance to die. Available from: www.gmc-uk.org/-/media/documents/gmc-guidance---when-a-patient-seeks-advice-or-information-about-assistance-to-die_pdf-61449907.pdf (accessed 16 January 2020).

27 Teed P. Access to medical records for assisted death: clarifying the guidance. Br J Gen Pract 2017; 67: 515.

28 Lewis P. The medical exception. CLP 2012; 65: 355–76.

29 *R v Brown (Anthony Joseph)* [1994] 1 AC 212.

30 Black I. Better off dead? Best interests assisted death [PhD thesis]. London: King's College London, 2016.

31 Arrhenius G, Rabinowicz W. The value of existence. In: Hirose I, Olson J, eds. The Oxford handbook of value theory. New York: Oxford University Press, 2015.

32 *State v Bass* (1961) 255 NC 42.

33 *Pretty v United Kingdom* (2002) 35 EHRR 1.

34 NHS, Blood and Transplant. Get the facts about organ donation. Available from: www.organdonation.nhs.uk/helping-you-to-decide/about-organ-donation/get-the-facts/ (accessed 16 January 2020).

Chapter 5: Assisted Dying in Canada: Lessons from the First 3 Years

Gary Rodin, Gilla Shapiro, Joshua Wales, Madeline Li

Introduction

The legalization of medical assistance in dying (MAID) in Canada, on 17 June 2016,[1] is a dramatic example of public empowerment in healthcare occurring in response to widespread societal support, but without the approval of any major medical organization. This departure from the absolute prohibition against the taking of life has occurred in Canada and some other developed nations in the context of an ageing and more secularized society in which personal autonomy is a pre-eminent value and in which there are increasing expectations of personal control over the circumstances of dying and medical assistance to achieve this end.[2,3]

MAID has become a prevalent practice in Canada, with varying degrees of integration into mainstream medical systems in the first 3 years since its inception. During this period, more than 7000 people in Canada chose to end their lives through assisted dying, representing approximately 1% of deaths in this country and almost 2% of cancer-related deaths. In some respects, Canadian MAID statistics mirror those in other jurisdictions, with almost two-thirds of requests for MAID coming from individuals with cancer.[4] The prevalence of assisted dying in Canada initially increased and then plateaued over the last year. The overall proportion of medically assisted deaths is at the lower end of the international range, which varies from 0.4% of deaths in Oregon to 4% of deaths in the Netherlands.[2,3]

There have been lessons learned and unresolved issues identified related to MAID in Canada. The latter include how soon before the end of life MAID should be delivered, whether it should be made available to mature minors and to the psychiatrically ill and whether it should be delivered based on an advance directive of patients who are no longer competent at the time of its delivery. This chapter addresses some of the challenges faced and lessons learnt over the first 3 years of this new medical practice in Canada, which may be of value to other jurisdictions where legalization of assisted dying is under consideration or being implemented.

The process of legalization in Canada

MAID was decriminalized in Canada on 6 February 2015, after the Supreme Court determined that it was unconstitutional to prohibit assisting the death of a competent adult who consented to the termination of life and had a grievous and irremediable illness, disease or disability that caused enduring, intolerable suffering.[5] In the ruling known as *Carter v Canada*,[5] one of the appellants was Lee Carter, a woman who was suffering from spinal stenosis and desired assisted death. The Supreme Court ruling in this case was considered to permit assisted dying for non-terminal conditions, although the language of bill C-14, the federal legislation that subsequently legalized MAID in Canada, specified criteria that are narrower than might have been suggested by this case (Box 5.1). In particular, the legislation requires that an individual's medical condition be 'incurable', in an 'advanced state of irreversible decline', and that 'natural death has become reasonably foreseeable'.[1] For many, this language suggested that MAID would be limited to cases of terminal illness and it was left open to the judgement of assessors to determine what constitutes

Box 5.1 Eligibility criteria for MAID in Canada.[1]

- A person may receive MAID only if they meet all the following criteria:
- they are eligible – or, but for any applicable minimum period of residence or waiting period, would be eligible – for health services funded by a government in Canada;
- they are at least 18 years of age and capable of making decisions with respect to their health;
- they have a grievous and irremediable medical condition, defined as:
  - having a serious and incurable illness, disease or disability,
  - being in an advanced state of irreversible decline in capability,
  - the illness, disease or disability or state of decline causes them enduring physical or psychological suffering that is intolerable to them and cannot be relieved under conditions that they consider acceptable, and
  - their natural death has become reasonably foreseeable, taking into account all of their medical circumstances, without a prognosis necessarily having been made as to the specific length of time that they have remaining;
- they have made a voluntary request for MAID that, in particular, was not made as a result of external pressure; and
- they give informed consent to receive MAID after having been informed of the means that are available to relieve their suffering, including palliative care.

the 'reasonably foreseeable) future. However, this judgement has not been as straightforward to clinicians making determinations for MAID as the legislators might have presumed.

The ambiguity in the legislation might have facilitated its acceptance by stakeholders with diverse views regarding eligibility, but it has also contributed to substantial variability in the interpretation and application of the law by MAID assessors and providers. The wording of the legislation allows MAID to be delivered in Canada to individuals with chronic medical conditions who may be expected to survive for many years. This contrasts with legislation in several US states and in the state of Victoria, Australia, which limits assisted dying to those with an expected survival of 6 months.[6,7]

The application of a broad definition of what is a 'reasonably foreseeable death) is similar in principle, if not in semantics, to other jurisdictions such as the Netherlands, where being 'tired of living) is an accepted indication for assisted dying.[8] Broader interpretations of the eligibility criteria in some regions may account for up to twofold variations in the rates of assisted dying varying across the provinces of Canada (Figure 5.1) and for the rate in some regions being 10 times greater than the national average.[9] MAID is currently being delivered in Canada to some patients who may be years from the end of life, although whether the framework and terminology that are applied in terminal illness are appropriate for chronic conditions is open to question.

The Supreme Court ruling held that suffering should be 'intolerable to the individual in the circumstances of his or her condition', and bill C-14 added 'physical or psychological suffering that is intolerable to them and that cannot be relieved under conditions that they consider acceptable'. This absolute reliance on the patient to establish what is intolerable suffering differs substantially

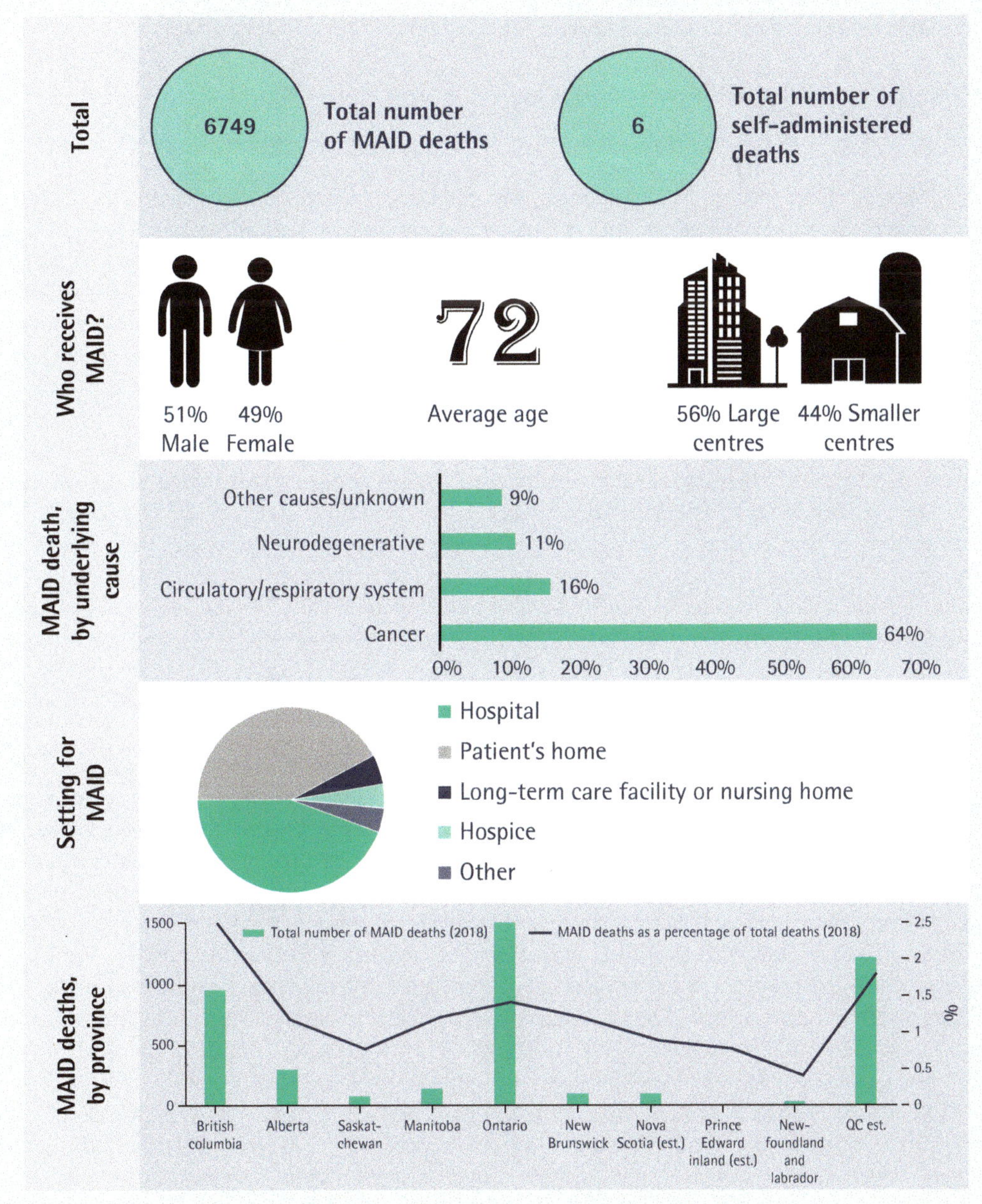

Figure 5.1 A snapshot of MAID in Canada. est., estimated.

from the assessment for other medical interventions, which are at least partly based on the judgement of clinicians. This complete reliance on the subjective report of patients to establish what is 'intolerable) suffering was intended to protect the legal rights of patients but can potentially override the perspective of clinicians. Further, the inclusion in this criterion of all forms of subjective suffering – physical or psychological – has contributed to the blurring of the boundary between intolerable suffering and being 'tired of living'.[10]

Protecting vulnerable populations

Attention was paid in the drafting of the MAID legislation in Canada to protecting the rights and safety of vulnerable individuals. Safeguards in this legislation include the mandate that there be two witnesses of the written MAID request who neither benefit from the individual's death nor provide direct personal care to the individual, two assessors who are independent of each other, and a 10 day waiting period after the signing of the MAID request, unless death or loss of capacity is imminent.[11] Further, an advance directive or substitute consent for MAID is not permitted, to protect vulnerable individuals who are no longer able to provide informed consent from having MAID imposed on them. Evidence that the desire for death can fluctuate widely, even in the last 2 weeks of life,[12] may justify the requirement that informed consent be obtained at the time of MAID delivery. However, the requirement that those requesting MAID be able to provide informed consent, not only at the time of the assessment but also at the time that it is delivered, has generated unintended distress for many eligible individuals and their caregivers. Those who have been approved for MAID may fear that they will lose competence and become ineligible for this intervention, forcing them to select a date to receive MAID that may be sooner than they would have otherwise chosen. In fact, recent data from a tertiary care centre indicate that the 10 day waiting period was shortened in almost 40% of cases approved for MAID because of concerns about the loss of capacity to provide informed consent.[13]

Mode of delivery and access to MAID

MAID legislation in Canada permits assisted dying both by means of oral ingestion of a prescribed medication and by intravenous injection performed by either a physician or a nurse practitioner. In practice, however, MAID in Canada has almost entirely been delivered in the form of clinician-administered intravenous injection (Figure 5.1). The preponderance of euthanasia was initially due to difficulties with the availability of oral secobarbital and to concern about the more variable logistical processes with oral administration. However, the greater predictability and reliability of intravenous injection and the value placed on the personal relationship between the patient and the healthcare provider in euthanasia may account for this ongoing predominant preference.

The right of healthcare providers to conscientiously object to participate in MAID is embedded in the Canadian Supreme Court ruling, although debate continues regarding the limits of this right. The College of Physicians and Surgeons of Ontario, the Canadian province with the highest absolute number of MAID deaths, ruled that all physicians were obliged to make an 'effective referral) for assessment of patients who requested this procedure.[14] Effective referral in this circumstance is defined as one provided 'in a timely manner to another physician, healthcare provider or agency who is non-objecting, accessible and available to the patient'.[15] There have been physicians who have objected to the requirement to make an effective referral for MAID or who have refused to participate in transplanting organs from patients who have died as a result of MAID.[16] However, there have been no sanctions thus far against physicians who refuse to make an effective referral or against institutions that do not provide MAID. MAID is currently not provided in many Canadian publicly funded faith-based healthcare facilities, even for hospitalized patients near the end of life. Access to MAID and many other medical services may also be limited in many rural and remote regions in Canada due to limitations in human resources and in healthcare systems.

Implementation and oversight

The process of implementing MAID in Canada did not involve a coordinated approach. Indeed, provinces and territories, medical institutions and individual clinicians were left to develop their own processes consistent with the legislation. A more systematic and coordinated framework would have been of particular value to community-based providers and to smaller institutions and communities, many of which experienced difficulty mobilizing sufficient resources to develop a rigorous process for the assessment and delivery of MAID. Jurisdictions implementing MAID would benefit from early consideration of how best to educate and support all healthcare providers and institutional staff with direct or indirect involvement in MAID. Such attention is essential to prepare all of those involved in or affected by MAID, in order to avoid misinformation, to protect the well-being of patients and providers, and to ensure rigour, consistency and efficiency in the process.

Oversight of individual MAID cases in Canada has also been left to individual provinces and territories, with no common national oversight regarding access to MAID or appropriateness of cases. MAID deaths are reported to and investigated by provincial and territorial offices of the chief coroner, chief medical examiners, ministries of health or designated MAID investigation units. Concerns about inappropriate practices are escalated to medical regulatory colleges, although investigations to date have related more to procedural issues than to substantive questions about the eligibility of cases. In the third year of MAID practice, the Canadian government instituted federal data collection on MAID processes,[17] but there is still no federal coordination of case reviews, such as that established in the Netherlands,[18] to ensure quality of care. A national approach of this kind would be of value to ensure rigour and a greater degree of consistency in the process of MAID assessment and delivery.

MAID and palliative care

The term palliative care was coined in 1975 by Balfour Mount, an early leader of palliative care in Canada.[19,20] Since that time, palliative care in Canada has grown to include a comprehensive network of home-based, ambulatory, hospital-based palliative care consultative services and inpatient units, and freestanding residential hospices. There are now two routes for physicians to obtain specialized training in palliative care. The College of Family Physicians of Canada offers a 'certificate of added competence in palliative care) for family physicians after an additional year of training, and the Royal College of Physicians and Surgeons of Canada provides specialty certification in palliative medicine through a 2 year programme followed by an exam. Specialized palliative care in Canada is widely available in many urban centres, particularly for patients with advanced cancer. However, there continue to be major gaps in palliative care services, particularly in rural and more remote regions. In that regard, a 2016–2017 report concluded that as few as 15% of people in Canada who could benefit from palliative care actually receive it.[21] Based on these findings, the Canadian government developed a 2018 framework on palliative care in order to improve the quality and universality of access to palliative care in Canada.[22]

Assisted dying has been as contentious a topic in the palliative care community in Canada as in other countries. A 2015 survey found that the majority of palliative care physicians in Canada do not approve of MAID,[23] and the Canadian Society of Palliative Care Physicians (CSPCP) firmly stated that it does not consider MAID to be an element of palliative care.[24] Their view is similar to that of many other American and European palliative care organizations.[25,26] In particular, the CSPCP has expressed concern that patients may choose MAID owing to a lack of access to palliative care that could otherwise ameliorate their suffering. They also noted that the intent of palliative care is to treat suffering, rather than to intentionally end life, and expressed fear that inclusion of MAID within palliative care would erode public trust in the field. Some in the field also expressed fear that the implementation of MAID would detract from efforts to increase access to palliative care.[27] That view has been challenged by evidence that the introduction of MAID has enhanced public attention to palliative and end of life care and that most patients who receive assisted dying also have access to palliative care in centres where it is readily available.[28,29]

Despite the contentious debate about MAID in the Canadian palliative care community, there is wide agreement on the importance of palliative care for patients and families before and after the administration of MAID. Most palliative care services and providers across Canada are not involved in the delivery of MAID, although there are examples of MAID provision being successfully integrated into palliative care services.[30] Most palliative care services and providers are involved in supporting patients and families through the process of MAID, from the time of initial consideration and decision making to before and after the actual delivery of MAID. While MAID can be provided by clinicians from diverse specialties, the unique expertise of palliative care providers has been especially valuable in MAID assessments and discussions, which often involve nuanced examination of suffering as well as explanations of available alternatives for end of life symptom management, including palliative sedation.

Conclusion

The experience of assisted dying in Canada indicates that an intervention such as MAID, which generated polarized and heated debate, can be implemented and normalized within a relatively short period of time. MAID continues to be facilitated and provided by physicians and nurse practitioners from diverse specialties, and robust professional organizations have emerged to support those involved in this activity. MAID has not been formally supported by palliative care organizations and bodies in Canada, but the assessment and delivery of MAID now occurs alongside palliative care and the process frequently involves palliative care physicians, nurses and settings. Further, the legalization and introduction of MAID may be seen to reflect the democratization of decision making in end of life care, which may be the most remarkable aspect of assisting dying in Canada and elsewhere.

The experience in Canada has highlighted the importance of a systemic and systematic approach to educating patients and all healthcare providers in the introduction of MAID and the need for national oversight and review of the practice. Ambiguity in the Canadian eligibility criteria for MAID might have initially diminished conflict among dissenting stakeholders and constituencies, but it has complicated the assessment process and limited the establishment of a clear standard of care. These challenges in interpreting the eligibility criteria have already generated several legal challenges. Other questions, such as whether MAID should be available to mature minors, to the psychiatrically ill or to those with an advance directive remain to be addressed.

End of life care in modern and more secularized societies has become a medicalized process in which healthcare providers are delegated the task of 'choreographing death'[31] and making it 'culturally meaningful'.[32] This must involve simultaneously attending to the rights of patients to receive this intervention and that of health professionals to conscientiously object to participation in it. There remain unresolved conflicts between these rights when physicians object to making effective referral for MAID or to participating in organ transplantation from patients who have died with MAID. Similar conflicts arise when healthcare institutions do not provide MAID for eligible consenting inpatients who are near the end of life and who cannot easily or safely be moved to another setting.

The legalization of MAID in Canada rapidly shifted the conversation in this country from whether to how MAID should be implemented. It is now clear that it can be made available without compromising palliative care and without abuse of the intervention. However, the central question of whether the legalization of MAID constitutes a net overall public good will require a longer period of time and diverse methodologies in order to evaluate it.[28]

Acknowledgement

The authors are grateful to Camilla Zimmermann for her constructive review of the manuscript and to Anne Rydall for her editorial assistance.

References

1 Statutes of Canada. Chapter 3. An Act to amend the criminal code and to make related amendments to other Acts (medical assistance in dying) (S.C. 2016, c.3). Assented to 2016–06–17 (bill C-14). Available from: https://laws-lois.justice.gc.ca/eng/annualstatutes/2016_3/fulltext.html (accessed 17 October 2019).

2 Eliott JA, Olver IN. Dying cancer patients talk about euthanasia. Soc Sci Med 2008; 67: 647–56.

3 Dowbiggen I. A merciful end: the euthanasia movement in modern America. New York: Oxford University Press, 2003.

4 Health Canada (2019). Fourth interim report on medical assistance in dying in Canada. Available from: www.canada.ca/en/health-canada/services/publications/health-system-services/medical-assistance-dying-interim-report-april-2019.html (accessed 17 October 2019).

5 *Carter v Canada (Attorney General).* Supreme Court judgments 2015 SCC 5 (2015–02–06; case 35591). Available from: https://scc-csc.lexum.com/scc-csc/scc-csc/en/item/14637/index.do (accessed 17 October 2019).

6 Emanuel EJ, Onwuteaka-Philipsen BD, Urwin JW, Cohen J. Attitudes and practices of euthanasia and physician-assisted suicide in the United States, Canada, and Europe. JAMA 2016; 316: 79–90.

7 Kirby T. Australian state of Victoria passes assisted dying bill. Lancet Respir Med 2018; 6: 182.

8 van Wijngaarden E, Goossensen A, Leget C. The social-political challenges behind the wish to die in older people who consider their lives to be completed and no longer worth living. J Eur Soc Policy 2018; 28: 419–29.

9 Robertson WD, Beuthin R. A review of medical assistance in dying on Vancouver Island: the first two years July 2016–July 2018. Available from: www.islandhealth.ca/sites/default/files/2018–11/maid-report-2016–2018.pdf (accessed 17 October 2019).

10 Florijn BW. Extending euthanasia to those 'tired of living) in the Netherlands could jeopardize a well-functioning practice of physicians) assessment of a patient's request for death. Health Policy 2018; 122: 315–19.

11 Downie J, Chandler JA, Institute for Research on Public Policy (2018). Interpreting Canada's medical assistance in dying legislation. Available from: https://on-irpp.org/2I7yQ6p (accessed 17 October 2019).

12 Rosenfeld B, Pessin H, Marziliano A, et al. Does desire for hastened death change in terminally ill cancer patients? Soc Sci Med 2014; 111: 35–40.

13 Selby D, Bean S, Isenberg-Grzeda E, et al. Medical assistance in dying (MAiD): a descriptive study from a Canadian tertiary care hospital. Am J Hosp Palliat Care 2020; 37: 58–64.

14 Trigg R. Conscientious objection and 'effective referral'. Camb Q Healthc Ethics 2017; 26: 32–43.

15 Government of Canada (2019). Medical assistance in dying. Available from: www.canada.ca/en/health-canada/services/medical-assistance-dying.html (accessed 17 October 2019).

16 Downar J, Shemie SD, Gillrie C, et al. Deceased organ and tissue donation after medical assistance in dying and other conscious and competent donors: guidance for policy. CMAJ 2019; 191: E604–13. [Erratum in: CMAJ 2019; 191: E745.]

17 Government of Canada (2018). Monitoring system for medical assistance in dying in Canada. Available from: www.canada.ca/en/health-canada/services/publications/health-system-services/monitoring-system-medical-assistance-dying.html (accessed 18 October 2019).

18 Miller DG, Kim SYH. Euthanasia and physician-assisted suicide not meeting due care criteria in the Netherlands: a qualitative review of review committee judgements. BMJ Open 2017; 7: e017628.

19 Lutz S. The history of hospice and palliative care. Curr Probl Cancer 2011; 35: 304–9.

20 Phillips D. Palliative Care McGill. Portraits: Balfour Mount. Available from: www.mcgill.ca/palliativecare/portraits-0/balfour-mount (accessed 18 October 2019).

21 Costante A, Lawand C, Cheng C. Access to palliative care in Canada. Healthc Q 2019; 21: 10–12.

22 Government of Canada (2018, modified 2019). Framework on palliative care in Canada. Available from: www.canada.ca/en/health-canada/services/health-care-system/reports-publications/palliative-care/framework-palliative-care-canada.html (accessed 18 October 2019).

23 Eggertson L. Most palliative physicians want no role in assisted death. CMAJ 2015; 187: E177.

24 Canadian Society of Palliative Care Physicians (2019). Updated key messages: palliative care and medical assistance in dying (MAID). Available from: www.cspcp.ca/category/medical-aid-in-dying-maid (accessed 18 October 2019).

25 American Academy of Hospice and Palliative Medicine (2016). Statement on physician-assisted dying. Available from: http://aahpm.org/positions/pad (accessed 18 October 2019).

26 Radbruch L, Leget C, Bahr P, et al. Euthanasia and physician-assisted suicide: a white paper from the European Association for Palliative Care. Palliat Med 2016; 30: 104–16.

27 Collins A, Leier B. Can medical assistance in dying harm rural and remote palliative care in Canada? Can Fam Physician 2017; 63: 186–90.

28 Li M, Watt S, Escaf M, et al. Medical assistance in dying – implementing a hospital-based program in Canada. N Engl J Med 2017; 376: 2082–8.

29 Dierickx S, Deliens L, Cohen J, Chambaere K. Involvement of palliative care in euthanasia practice in a context of legalized euthanasia: a population-based mortality follow-back study. Palliat Med 2017; 32: 114–22.

30 Wales J, Isenberg SR, Wegier P, et al. Providing medical assistance in dying within a home palliative care program in Toronto, Canada: an observational study of the first year of experience. J Palliat Med 2018; 21: 1573–9.

31 Buchbinder M. Choreographing death: a social phenomenology of medical aid-in-dying in the United States. Med Anthropol Q 2018; 32: 481–97.

32 Timmermans S. Death brokering: constructing culturally appropriate deaths. Sociol Health Illn 2005; 27: 993–1013.

Chapter 6: Provision of Palliative Care in the UK: How does the Research Evidence Compare with Current Practice?

Andrew Page, Michael I. Bennett

Introduction

In the UK, cancer accounted for 28.1% of all 533,000 deaths registered in 2017 and has remained the most common broad cause of death since 2011.[1] Between the ages of 55 and 70, cancer accounts for half of all female deaths and between 35% and 45% of all male deaths. Circulatory diseases such as heart disease and stroke were the second most common broad cause of death, accounting for 25% of all deaths registered in 2017, followed by respiratory diseases, which accounted for 13.8%.[1] By 2041, it is predicted that the number of people aged over 85 years will double from 1.6 million to 3.2 million[2] and will account for 56% of the predicted palliative care need.[3] Estimates suggest that by 2040 there will be at least a 25% increase in all deaths, largely driven by cancer (143,000 deaths in 2017 to 208,000 deaths in 2040) and dementia among this ageing demographic.[3]

The World Health Organization defines palliative care as: 'An approach that improves the quality of life of patients and their families facing the problems associated with life-threatening illness ... Palliative care is applicable early in the course of illness, in conjunction with other therapies that are intended to prolong life.'[4] Key components of palliative care involve pain and symptom control, psychosocial support and advance care planning,[4] which form the basis of a specialist palliative care consultation. Symptom burden varies substantially between diagnoses, but common symptomatology exists in a palliative care cohort.[5] Fatigue (13–100%), pain (11–94%), anorexia (13–95%), dyspnoea (11–98%) and worry (3–86%) have been highlighted as the most commonly occurring palliative care symptoms across cancer and non-cancer groups, with fatigue being the most prevalent at the end of life.[5] Palliative care patients generally suffer a multitude (median five) of complex and ever-changing symptoms,[6] some of which directly or indirectly (e.g. via therapeutic intervention) impact each other. A patient-centred approach prioritizes the most debilitating symptoms for each patient, balancing achievable symptom control with side effects. For example, a patient with pain and fatigue may prefer suboptimal pain control to avoid increasing fatigue.

Despite current symptom management strategies, certain symptoms remain intractable and often progressive despite correction of contributory reversible components. Disability, debility and increasing dependence, commonly linked with a feeling of loss of dignity,[7] are examples of such challenging and often insurmountable symptoms. Open discussions about what is realistically achievable for patients remains a cornerstone of the palliative care approach.

This chapter highlights the provision of palliative care in the UK and discusses the gap that exists between research evidence and what patients experience in routine care, particularly in relation to important outcomes towards the end of life.

Palliative care in the UK

A 2016 qualitative study reported by the British Medical Association (BMA) highlighted the importance of a palliative care approach for all patients with advanced progressive disease.[8] The BMA asked the public and doctors what most concerned them about end of life and dying, and the commonest concerns for both groups were pain, followed by impact on loved ones, being a burden, loss of dignity, and poor care or continuity of care.

The development of hospices and palliative care services began in the UK in the 1970s. Services are now widespread, making the UK the world leader in the palliative care rankings of the Quality of Death Index compiled by The Economist Intelligence Unit.[9] National policy in the UK to improve end of life care began in 2008 with the publication of the Department for Health's end of life care strategy, updated in 2015 to the National Ambitions for Palliative and End of Life Care.[10] These advocate person-centred care and early recognition of those who may benefit from palliative care support. Even in the UK, however, the geographical provision of palliative care services varies widely.[11]

Alongside the development of palliative care in the last 40 years, there have been substantial changes in the treatment of some cancers, resulting in significant improvements in survival rates. For example, common cancers such as breast, prostate, colorectal and kidney have seen 30–40% increases in 5 year survival rates.[12] By contrast, however, the overall survival of patients with cancers of lung, stomach, pancreas and oesophagus has changed very little in this time. As some cancers are now regarded as chronic diseases, recognizing the palliative and terminal phases of these illnesses has become more difficult. The challenge of prognostication, like in non-cancer patients, is an important factor in palliative care access.[13]

Evidence of efficacy of palliative care

Recently published meta-analyses of randomized clinical trials, mostly in cancer patients, have shown benefits of integrating palliative care support before death, but the outcomes are nuanced.[14–20] Overall, palliative care support improves quality of life but the effect size is small.[17–20] Benefits on pain and symptom management are inconclusive: three meta-analyses showed no evidence of improvement,[15,17,18] while another suggested reduced symptom intensity overall but not for pain specifically.[19] Other reported effects include increased chance of home death, reduced hospitalization at the end of life, and no effect on survival.[15–19]

In general terms, the trials included in these meta-analyses recruited patients at the time of diagnosis of advanced disease (around 6–12 months before death) and provided several assessments by multidisciplinary teams over a period of 3–4 months. This promoted a recommendation that, for full benefits of palliative care to be realized, continuity by a multidisciplinary team was needed for at least 3–4 months (before death).[21]

In 2012, the American Society of Clinical Oncology issued guidance to its members recommending, 'Palliative care should be considered early in the course of illness for any patient with metastatic cancer and/or high symptom burden.'[22] There has been debate about when referral is optimal and what might prompt referral. Recommendations include referral to be made within 3 months of diagnosis of advanced cancer or progressive disease, combined with an assessment of needs.[23]

However, not all trials of earlier integration of palliative care in cancer patients have shown benefits.[24–27] Even in 'positive' trials, differential responses are apparent. One example is the large randomized controlled trial reported by Temel et al.,[28] which recruited patients with advanced lung and upper gastrointestinal (GI) cancers. The intervention had significant effects on quality of life and mood for the combined sample, but sensitivity analysis revealed that benefits were experienced by lung cancer patients only and not upper GI cancer patients.

Data from these 'negative) trials are important to weigh up against previous 'positive) trials, because the evidence suggests that not every patient with advanced cancer benefits from earlier palliative care. Equally, from a service perspective, it is unlikely to be cost-effective to provide this early support to all patients. It also seems likely that patients with needs (which generally increase closer to death) are more likely to benefit than those without clear needs despite having advanced cancer. Perhaps needs-based referral triggers are more important than time-based referral triggers.

Access to palliative care

Each year in the UK, about 200,000 people receive some form of support from palliative care services.[29] This is commonly in the form of advice and management from community- or hospital-based nurse specialist teams but may also include medical outpatient consultations or inpatient admission for more intensive symptom management or end of life care by multidisciplinary teams.

Even in well-resourced countries such as the UK and USA, service provision is far from ideal.[13,30,31] Historical links between palliative care and oncology, and the challenges of identifying terminal phases of non-cancer diseases, have meant that there is often inequality of access to palliative care services. The UK National Survey of Bereaved People (Views of Informal Carers – Evaluation of Services, VOICES) asks randomly sampled bereaved relatives who registered a death to provide details of their loved one's illness and care in last 3 months of life. Analysis of pooled data between 2011 and 2015 for patients who had been cared for at home, and which excluded sudden death, found that in the 50% of deaths caused by cancer, 62.7% of these patients had received some palliative care support before they died. This contrasts with only 9.9% of the remaining half of patients who received palliative care support before they died from non-cancer diseases.[32] Increasing access for non-cancer patients remains a key aim of the national end of life strategy in the UK and has helped to increase non-cancer referrals from 5% in 2000 to 20% in 2013.[10,33,34] A cancer diagnosis remains, however, the main determinant of access to palliative care services,[33,35] despite evidence that non-cancer patients suffer from a similar symptom burden.[5,36] However, a cancer diagnosis is not a guarantee of receiving specialist palliative care. Underrepresented cancer patients are older, male, have lung cancer, have not received an opioid prescription or have not received chemotherapy.[37]

For patients who do access palliative care, what is the duration of this support before death? The research evidence described above suggests that 3–4 months (12–16 weeks) of palliative care before death is optimal. A national UK analysis of nearly 43,000 deaths within palliative care services in 2015 showed that the median interval between referral and death was 48 days (7 weeks); 40% of patients were referred within 4 weeks of their death.[38] Patients with cancer received twice the duration of support compared with non-cancer patients (53 days vs 27 days). However, regardless of underlying disease, patients over 75 years of age received about half the duration of palliative care compared with younger patients (39 days vs 78 days).

Given this gap between research evidence and clinical practice in relation to access and duration of palliative care, is there evidence of improved patient outcomes in routine data? A study in 2479 patients who died of cancer in one UK city linked primary and secondary care records for the last year of life.[39] Decedents who received palliative care were significantly more likely to die in a hospice (39.4% vs 14.5%) and less likely to die in hospital (23.3% vs 40.1%); palliative care initiated more than 2 weeks before death was associated with avoiding a hospital death; more than 4 weeks before death was associated with avoiding emergency hospital admissions.

The Department for Health's end of life care strategy aims to enable people to die in their preferred place, which is commonly thought for most to be their home.[10] However, do patients actually want to die at home? A systematic review conducted by Hoare et al.[40] found that only 40% of patients wanted to die at home, compared with 63% of the general public surveyed when missing data of preferences were taken into account. Interestingly, the review also found that only 27% of families would want their relative to die at home. This highlights how families can be a poor proxy for a patient's preferred place of death, with implications for UK health policy that relies heavily on next-of-kin advocacy.[40] Caution should be taken in assuming home should be the default location of future care for dying patients, particularly those who are currently being cared for in other settings.

Palliative care and pain control

Given the importance of pain control to patients facing the end of life, as well as to carers and healthcare professionals,[8] it is surprising that evidence from meta-analyses does not support an important effect of palliative care support on improving pain outcomes.[15–19] However, it is important to highlight that pain was not the primary outcome of these meta-analyses or the research they included, and studies were relatively small. Comparatively, the VOICES survey data sampled opinion from a more than 10-fold sample size, which demonstrated that pain control in the last 3 months of life was completely or almost completely controlled in 86.6% of patients within a hospice setting, compared with care homes (73.6%), hospitals (68.4%) or home (48.6%),[32] despite the complexity of patients who frequent inpatient palliative care units.

Equally, the meta-analyses) findings might be partly explained because patients with advanced cancer often receive strong opioids late in their disease process. Studies show that less than half of all cancer patients who die in the UK and Canada receive a strong opioid before death,[41–43] and in those who received opioids the median treatment initiation was 9 weeks prior to death.[41] In routine care, cancer patients who access palliative care are far more likely to be prescribed a strong opioid before death than those who are not referred (53% vs 25.2%; $p<0.001$), and increased duration of palliative care is associated with increasing odds of receiving a strong opioid.[39] This suggests that access to palliative care does lead to improved pain management. This is further corroborated by analysis of the VOICES data that showed that cancer patients who received palliative care support at home were much more likely to experience good pain relief compared with those who did not (67% vs 39%).[32] Regression models found that good pain relief was 2.67 times more likely when patients received specialist palliative care.

Conclusion

 The UK is a world leader in palliative care provision, and research evidence demonstrates overall important benefits for patients who access such care. However, in routine care, access and duration of palliative care are not equitable and for most cancer patients are limited, with research suggesting they receive it for less than the 3–4 months required to achieve optimal benefits. Nevertheless, even shorter durations of palliative care (at least 4 weeks) can be associated with significant benefits, including significantly improved pain control. Patients with non-cancer diagnoses remain underrepresented in both research and their ability to access palliative care services. Routine screening for palliative care needs and using it to trigger referral for palliative care support seem the most equitable way of providing end of life support for patients in the future.

References

1 Office for National Statistics (2017). Deaths registered in England and Wales: 2017. Available from: www.ons.gov.uk/peoplepopulationandcommunity/birthsdeathsandmarriages/deaths/bulletins/deathsregistrationsummarytables/2017 (accessed 10 September 2019).

2 Office for National Statistics (2016). National population projections: 2016-based statistical bulletin. Available from: www.ons.gov.uk/peoplepopulationandcommunity/populationandmigration/populationprojections/bulletins/nationalpopulationprojections/2016basedstatisticalbulletin (accessed 10 September 2019).

3 Etkind SN, Bone AE, Gomes B, et al. How many people will need palliative care in 2040? Past trends, future projections and implications for services. BMC Med 2017; 15: 102.

4 World Health Organization. WHO definition of palliative care. Available from: www.who.int/cancer/palliative/definition/en (accessed 10 September 2019).

5 Moens K, Higginson IJ, Harding R. Are there differences in the prevalence of palliative care-related problems in people living with advanced cancer and eight non-cancer conditions? A systematic review. J Pain Symptom Manage 2014; 48: 660–77.

6 Oechsle K, Goerth K, Bokemeyer C, Mehnert A. Symptom burden in palliative care patients: perspectives of patients, their family caregivers, and their attending physicians. Support Care Cancer 2013; 21: 1955–62.

7 Woo JA, Maytal G, Stern TA. Clinical challenges to the delivery of end-of-life care. Prim Care Companion J Clin Psychiatry 2006; 8: 367–72.

8 British Medical Association (2016, updated 2018). End-of-life care and physician-assisted dying. Available from: www.bma.org.uk/collective-voice/policy-and-research/ethics/end-of-life-care (accessed 10 September 2019).

9 The Economist Intelligence Unit (2015). The 2015 Quality of Death Index. Ranking palliative care across the world. Available from: https://eiuperspectives.economist.com/healthcare/2015-quality-death-index (accessed 10 September 2019).

10 National Palliative and End of Life Care Partnership (2015). Ambitions for palliative and end of life care: a national framework for local action 2015–2020. Available from: http://endoflifecareambitions.org.uk (accessed 10 September 2019).

11 Public Health England (2018). Atlas of variation for palliative and end of life care in England. Available from: https://fingertips.phe.org.uk/profile/atlas-of-variation (accessed 10 September 2019).

12 Quaresma M, Coleman MP, Rachet B. 40-year trends in an index of survival for all cancers combined and survival adjusted for age and sex for each cancer in England and Wales, 1971–2011: a population-based study. Lancet 2015; 385: 1206–18.

13 Dixon J, King D, Matosevic T, et al. (2015). Equity in the provision of palliative care in the UK: review of evidence. Available from: www.pssru.ac.uk/publication-details.php?id=4962 (accessed 10 September 2019).

14 Higginson IJ, Finlay IG, Goodwin DM, et al. Is there evidence that palliative care teams alter end-of-life experiences of patients and their caregivers? J Pain Symptom Manage 2003; 25: 150–68.

15 Gomes B, Calanzani N, Curiale V, et al. Effectiveness and cost-effectiveness of home palliative care services for adults with advanced illness and their caregivers. Cochrane Database Syst Rev 2013; 6: 1–279.

16 Luckett T, Davidson PM, Lam L, et al. Do community specialist palliative care services that provide home nursing increase rates of home death for people with life-limiting illnesses? A

systematic review and meta-analysis of comparative studies. J Pain Symptom Manage 2013; 45: 279–97.

17 Kavalieratos D, Corbelli J, Zhang D, et al. Association between palliative care and patient and caregiver outcomes: a systematic review and meta-analysis. JAMA 2016; 316: 2104–14.

18 Gaertner J, Siemens W, Meerpohl JJ, et al. Effect of specialist palliative care services on quality of life in adults with advanced incurable illness in hospital, hospice, or community settings: systematic review and meta-analysis. BMJ 2017; 357: j2925.

19 Haun MW, Estel S, Rücker G, et al. Early palliative care for adults with advanced cancer. Cochrane Database Syst Rev 2017; 6: CD011129.

20 Kassianos AP, Ioannou M, Koutsantoni M, Charalambous H. The impact of specialized palliative care on cancer patients) health-related quality of life: a systematic review and meta-analysis. Support Care Cancer 2018; 26: 61–79.

21 Davis MP, Temel JS, Balboni T Glare P. A review of the trials which examine early integration of outpatient and home palliative care for patients with serious illnesses. Ann Palliat Med 2015; 4: 99–121.

22 Smith TJ, Temin S, Alesi ER, et al. American Society of Clinical Oncology provisional clinical opinion: the integration of palliative care into standard oncology care. J Clin Oncol 2012; 30: 880–7.

23 Hui D, Mori M, Watanabe SM, et al. Referral criteria for outpatient specialty palliative cancer care: an international consensus. Lancet Oncol 2016; 17: e552–9.

24 Nordly M, Skov Benthien K, Vadstrup ES, et al. Systematic fast-track transition from oncological treatment to dyadic specialized palliative home care: DOMUS – a randomized clinical trial. Palliat Med 2019; 33: 135–49.

25 Groenvold M, Petersen MA, Damkier A, et al. Randomised clinical trial of early specialist palliative care plus standard care versus standard care alone in patients with advanced cancer: the Danish Palliative Care Trial. Palliat Med 2017; 31: 814–24.

26 Brims F, Gunatilake S, Lawrie I, et al. Early specialist palliative care on quality of life for malignant pleural mesothelioma: a randomised controlled trial. Thorax 2019; 74: 354–61.

27 Franciosi V, Maglietta G, Degli Esposti C, et al. Early palliative care and quality of life of advanced cancer patients – a multicenter randomized clinical trial. Ann Palliat Med 2019; 8: 381–9.

28 Temel JS, Greer JA, El-Jawahri A, et al. Effects of early integrated palliative care in patients with lung and GI cancer: a randomized clinical trial. J Clin Oncol 2017; 35: 834–41.

29 Hospice UK (2016). Hospice care in the UK 2016. Available from: www.hospiceuk.org/docs/default-source/What-We-Offer/publications-documents-and-files/hospice-care-in-the-uk-2016.pdf (accessed 10 September 2019).

30 Lancaster H, Finlay I, Downman M, Dumas J. Commissioning of specialist palliative care services in England. BMJ Support Palliat Care 2018; 8: 93–101.

31 Meier DE. Increased access to palliative care and hospice services: opportunities to improve value in healthcare. Milbank Q 2011; 89: 343–80.

32 El Mokhallalati Y, Woodhouse N, Farragher T, Bennett MI. Specialist palliative care support is associated with improved pain relief at home during last 3 months of life in patients with advanced disease: analysis of 5-year data from the National Survey of Bereaved People (VOICES). BMC Med 2019; 17: 50.

33 National Council for Palliative Care (2014). National survey of patient activity data for specialist palliative care services. Minimum data set for 2012–13. Available from: www.

endoflifecare-intelligence.org.uk/resources/publications/mdsreport2014 (archived) (accessed 10 September 2019).

34 National Council for Palliative Care (2012). National survey of patient activity data for specialist palliative care services. Minimum data set for 2010–11. Available from: www.endoflifecare-intelligence.org.uk/resources/publications/mds_report (archived) (accessed 10 September 2019).

35 Grande GE, Farquhar MC, Barclay SIG, Todd CJ. The influence of patient and carer age in access to palliative care services. Age Ageing 2006; 35: 267–73.

36 Solano JP, Gomes B, Higginson IJ. A comparison of symptom prevalence in far advanced cancer, AIDS, heart disease, chronic obstructive pulmonary disease and renal disease. J Pain Symptom Manage 2006; 31: 58–69.

37 Craigs C, West R, Hurlow A, et al. Access to palliative care for patients with advanced cancer: a longitudinal population analysis. PLoS One 2018; 13: e0200071.

38 Allsop MJ, Ziegler LE, Mulvey MR, et al. Duration and determinants of hospice-based specialist palliative care for patients in the UK. A national retrospective cohort study. Palliat Med 2018; 32: 1322–33.

39 Ziegler L, Craigs C, West R, et al. Is palliative care support associated with better quality end of life care indicators for patients with advanced cancer? A retrospective cohort study. BMJ Open 2018; 8: e018284.

40 Hoare S, Morris ZS, Kelly MP, et al. Do patients want to die at home? a systematic review of the UK literature, focused on missing preferences for place of death. PLoS One 2015; 10: e0142723.

41 Ziegler LE, Mulvey MR, Blenkinsopp A, et al. Opioid prescribing for cancer patients in the last year of life: a longitudinal population cohort study. Pain 2016; 157: 2445–51.

42 Higginson IJ, Gao W. Opioid prescribing for cancer pain during the last 3 months of life: associated factors and 9-year trends in a nationwide United Kingdom cohort study. J Clin Oncol 2012; 30: 4373–9.

43 Gagnon B, Scott S, Nadeau L, Lawlor PG. Patterns of community-based opioid prescriptions in people dying of cancer. J Pain Symptom Manage 2015; 49: 36–44.

Chapter 7: A palliative Care Perspective on Choices for End of Life Care in Cancer Patients

Rob George, Amy Proffitt

Introduction

People are free to commit suicide and refuse any treatment even when it will lead to an early death, but whether they should have the right to an assisted suicide or euthanasia is both contentious and political. The arguments are obscured by euphemism and ambiguity. We refer to providing the means for someone to commit suicide as 'assisted suicide) and anyone taking lethal action at the request of a person as 'administering euthanasia'. If either involves a doctor we use the terms 'physician-assisted suicide) or 'physician-administered euthanasia'. We do not comment on the rights and wrongs of suicide and euthanasia but confine our view to whether medicine should be involved. Most doctors working in palliative care do not support a change in the law.

Among other things, palliative care specializes in mitigating symptoms, managing the uncertainties of dying and relieving the suffering it may entail for patients and families. The emotional journey for them, and staff, may be so charged and tangled that distinguishing whose distress is uppermost at different stages is often difficult. Because death is the universal outcome, it is easy also to confuse intervention to control symptoms with altering the dying process: for example, to ascribe death soon after an injection (irrespective of the drug or its purpose) to that injection and not the underlying disease; or that a loved one not eating or drinking means death was from starvation or dehydration rather than from their cancer.

As clinicians we need to be very clear about what we are, and are not, doing in care as someone dies. This does not need special wisdom, but common sense and clarity about what is happening. We must be precise and factual, keeping clear our ethical or moral distinctions as we make judgements and take clinical action. In this chapter, we consider the facts, the potential risks and harms of certain actions, and the difference between suicide and expecting someone else to assist in it.

Factual considerations

Facts involve statements about what and how things are. They can differ in type or vary in degree. A cat and dog are different types of mammal, whereas it is a matter of degree when a mound becomes a hill and a hill becomes a mountain.

Is stopping a life-sustaining treatment the same as ending a life?

This section briefly covers why discontinuing or not offering potentially life-sustaining treatments is not physician-assisted suicide or euthanasia. The reason is that they are different types of action, i.e. they are factually different. Figure 7.1 depicts the following:

1 A causal chain begins when a disease initiates a sequence of events that left untreated will lead to death.

2 A diagnosis is made and treatment started.

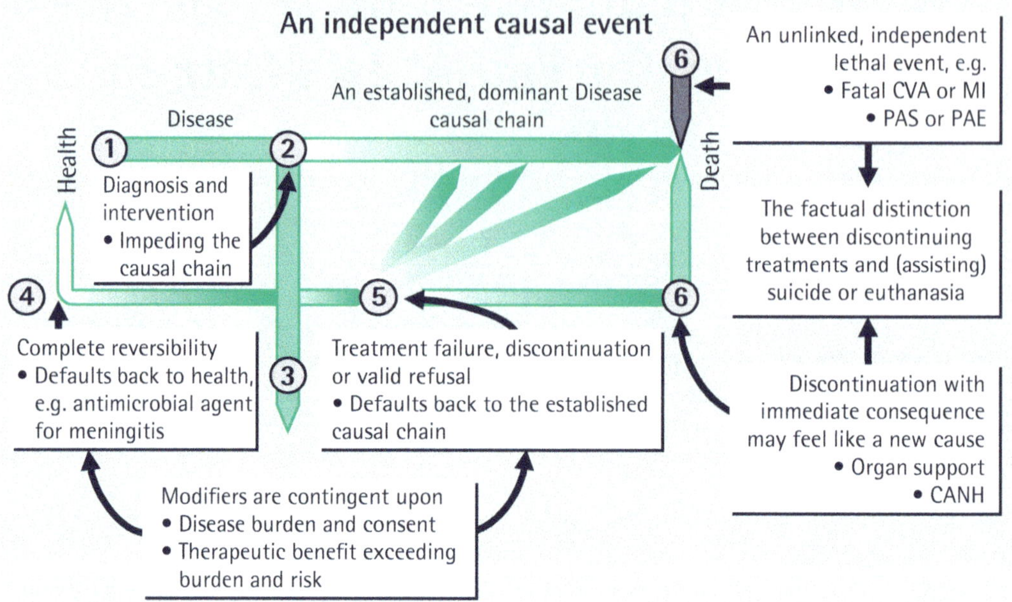

Figure 7.1 A diagrammatical expression of causation. CANH, clinically assisted nutrition and hydration; CVA, cerebrovascular accident; MI, myocardial infarction; PAE, physician-administered euthanasia; PAS, physician-assisted suicide.

3 Whether a treatment (modifier) should be given is contingent upon disease burden and therapeutic benefit exceeding burden, or risk and consent.

4 On the one hand, an entirely reversible trigger, such as an acute bacterial infection, can be aborted easily and ends the chain without iatrogenic consequence, so the person is back to full health.

5 The relevant trigger for us is a cancer +/− comorbidities acting alone or in concert, to drive the person towards death. Treatments (contingent modifiers) will impede this chain according to their efficacy, the aggregate burden of disease, its curability and whether the person consents to treatment.

6 At some point treatments will stop because of a combination of their failing or their burden or risk becoming intolerable and/or the person withdrawing consent. At that point the progression of pathology defaults back to the established causal chain of pathology and the person dies.

  – The speed with which that happens is determined by the causal gradient of the cumulative disease and treatment burden.

  – Removing the contingent modifiers does not bring about the death: it removes impediments to it (or indeed it may prolong life if the treatments came with significant burden and risk).

7 In situations where the initial insult has stabilized and life is sustained by organ support, such as ventilation, the unimpeded causal power is so great that removal leads rapidly to death (albeit in proportion to residual organ function) and feels emotionally like a life-ending act when it is not.[1] Equally, in a person with a disorder of consciousness, in which he or she is clinically stable

yet 'would be dead but for) clinically assisted nutrition, cessation also may feel like euthanasia when it is not.

- We stop treatments to avoid continued harm, not to precipitate death, even though we may not be obstructing it; points 5 and 6 are differences of degree within the same category. The law is very clear on this.

- In *Aintree University Hospitals NHS Foundation Trust v James*,[2] judging an application to withhold a number of life-sustaining treatments, the Supreme Court set out the principle governing continuing treatments: 'The fundamental question is whether it is in the patient's best interests, and therefore lawful, to give the treatment – not whether it is lawful to withhold it.'

8 A new causal chain is different because it is factually distinct, i.e. it is a categorical difference in type, not degree.

- An unexpected, unlinked fatal cerebral or cardiac event is clearly a discrete pathological cause in its own right.

- The decision to ingest or have prescribed or administered a lethal cocktail of drugs is an independent act.

Stopping treatments, suicide and physician-assisted suicide/euthanasia are not on a continuum as some claim. Palliative care physicians are clear that they are not 'already doing this all the time'.[3]

Two other largely factual questions remain.

Is assisting suicide different from administering euthanasia?

If one judges that a person needs an antibiotic for an infection, but he or she is unable to swallow, one would not hesitate to administer it by injection. This is a practical matter of fact about the degree of intervention. The ethical decision is whether the person should have an antibiotic in the first place. Canada is a legislature where lethal drugs are supplied to assist a suicide; if the person cannot swallow, administering euthanasia by injection is the practical solution. Physician-assisted suicide and physician-administered euthanasia are defined collectively as medical assistance in dying. It is nonsensical and disingenuous to distinguish them.[4] For palliative care, this means two things: that we consider the prescribing and administering of lethal drugs to be the same, and that data from all legislatures permitting physician-assisted suicide with or without physician-administered euthanasia are relevant when considering the inherent impact on and risks for patients and society in changing the law.

Can legislation justify limiting availability to certain groups?

This is both a factual and a moral issue. Attempts at legislation in the UK have always limited physician-assisted suicide to adults with mental capacity who are not mentally ill and who have a life-expectancy of less than 6 months. These sound like clear, factual categories, but all are differences of degree and therefore present practical problems of reliable assessment and qualification. Arbitrary boundaries are quickly and understandably crossed in all permissive legislatures.[5–7]

The moral ground is much clearer: if assisted suicide/euthanasia is legal for anyone, unjustifiable discrimination will prevent its being confined for long to those who have mental capacity and are dying, have life-limiting disease(s) and are adults.[4,8] All legislatures, including those in Oregon and Canada, clearly show this.[9,10]

We leave further discussion to one side. The spread of literature and commentary can be found at the online resource of the Association for Palliative Medicine of Great Britain and Ireland (APM).[11]

Moral/ethical considerations

Ethics and morals are interchangeable terms. They are the values one applies to the facts that enable a decision to be made and the right action taken. They are the language of interests that use words such as 'best', 'worst', 'benefits', 'burdens', 'risks) and 'harms'. Every action requires us first to apply values to weigh up the facts. Our personal ethic reflects the values that we hold as individuals; as professionals we must adhere to duties of care that comprise the values of medicine as laid out by the General Medical Council: cardinal among these are to avoid harm, act in a patient's best interests, and default in favour of life. These must underpin our motivations and intentions in offering, initiating or continuing treatments and in balancing benefits and harms.

Intent, responsibility and culpability: the compass of double effect

The road between risking unintended death from a treatment meant to benefit life and continuing to offer or deliver treatments with a small chance of buying days or weeks, knowing they may harm or shorten what life remains, is every doctor's concern. Double effect is the compass that helps us navigate this. It has five elements or tests (Box 7.1), discussed in detail elsewhere.[12] Double effect applies especially to specialties such as oncology in which treatments have narrow therapeutic ratios and substantial risks of grave or mortal harm. It seldom applies to palliative care but is always associated with it and with the mistaken claim that doctors kill patients regularly with opioids and sedation at the end of life.[13]

Involving doctors directly in physician-assisted suicide/euthanasia reframes 'benefits', 'harms) and 'interests) fundamentally, along with a new 'duty of care) for the responsible doctor of an eligible person to end life at that person's request. It also turns double effect on its head.

Benefits, harms and interests

Best interests go beyond medicine to incorporate the patient's welfare and what he or she regards as a life worth living. The Supreme Court in *Aintree University Hospitals NHS Foundation Trust v James*[2] defined 'best interests) as follows:

- 'Where a patient is suffering from an incurable illness, disease or disability, the prospects for success of a given treatment should be considered in respect of a return to a quality of life that the patient would regard as worthwhile.'

- 'The purpose of the best interests test is to consider matters from the patient's point of view. That is not to say that his wishes must prevail, any more than those of a fully capable patient must prevail. We cannot always have what we want. But insofar as it is possible to ascertain the patient's wishes, feelings, beliefs and values, it is those that should be taken into account in making the choice for him as an individual human being.'

Box 7.1 The five tests of a defensible double effect.[12]

- The intended act itself is good or at least indifferent.
- The bad effect is not a means to the good effect.
- The good effect, and not the bad effect (while foreseeable), is intended.
- (Importantly) the justification(s) for risking the bad effect should be proportionate in medicine, particularly in drug titrations that lead to unacceptable organ toxicities.[14]
- The agents minimize the foreseen harm, even if it involves accepting additional risk or foregoing some benefit.

Palliative care prides itself on trying explicitly to prioritize what matters to the person, and not just what the matter is with the person. We may not be able to buy time but we can help to buy quality. Good joint decision making balances threats to interests and it judges the wisdom of treatments that may harm. Put simply, a 'harm) is anything that has an adverse effect on our interests. Embracing this, and ensuring that what is on offer is considered in that light, may lead to unexpected plans. In this light the request of a young mother, insisting on involvement in a phase I study to try and buy any chance of additional time, only justifies support so long as she and the family know explicitly that the opposite may happen because of toxicities, and what time, if any, that is bought may be of very poor quality or spent in hospital. Alternatively, decisions to forego a treatment early through fears of side effects when symptoms may benefit as much as survival need to be approached with equal honesty. Candour is a duty not just when things go wrong, but in order to anticipate and engage the risk of bad outcomes as part of consent. This is the heart of conversations on consent. Figure 7.2 summarizes the interrelationship between benefits and harms, which is the substrate of discussion and review of someone's goals of treatment:

1 At diagnosis of an incurable malignancy, one would expect treatment to produce some improvement in health but ultimately a decline and death (denoted by the dashed line and palest shading).

2 There will be accompanying burdens or potential harms from treatment (denoted by the dotted-dashed line and dark shading) that frequently fall once intense treatments end.

3 If treatment continues or changes when health deteriorates, the harms will ultimately rise.

4 At an individualized point the aggregate burdens will cease to be acceptable and a decision made to stop treatment.

5 It is hoped that the burdens associated with treatment will fall.

6 Those who are frail, have multiple morbidities or have been diagnosed very late often present a very finely balanced set of pros and cons as to the aggregated benefit or harm of intervention.

7 They may never have treatments or will tolerate them less and stop them earlier.

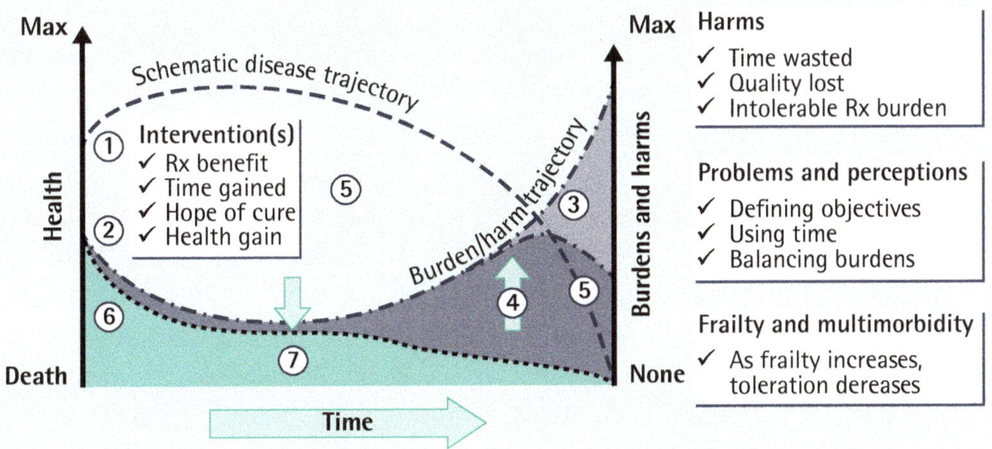

Figure 7.2 The interrelationship between benefits and harms. Rx, treatment.

The most precious commodity for a dying person is time, but time with quality. To waste a dying person's time is wrong. Exhausting journeys to hospital for fruitless appointments, unnecessary tests or hollow promises of cure/biological stability – at the expense of the chance to complete key tasks, repair and enrich relationships or resolve issues – are the harms to personal interests to which the Supreme Court's ruling in *Aintree University Hospitals NHS Foundation Trust v James* points.[2]

Is there, however, a limit in deferring to personal interest: is judging a life harmful, considering or agreeing that a person would be better off dead and offering death as a treatment in the proper domain of medicine? The fact that having access to assisted suicide/euthanasia may be a good idea is a question for society that is independent of who is expected to do it. The issue here is whether it should be a part of medicine, i.e. a treatment and a potential duty of care, which is entirely separate. International evidence shows it to be uncontainable when in the hands of doctors.[12] The vast majority of those practising palliative medicine believe that it should not be part of healthcare at all.

This brings us to the extent and limits of an individual's freedoms and entitlements to realize his or her interests, i.e. the individual's autonomy.

Autonomy

Autonomy is how interests are expressed. In a medico-legal sense, it is relatively black and white: we are free to realize our interests, even to harm ourselves, so long as it does not harm others. In a social sense, it is much more complex, because we are relational and every action unavoidably affects those around us to some extent. Autonomy is not a *carte blanche*: it is about limits, not just liberties. As the Supreme Court reminded us in *Aintree University Hospitals NHS Foundation Trust v James*: 'The purpose of the best interests test is to consider matters from the patient's point of view. That is not to say that his wishes must prevail, any more than those of a fully capable patient must prevail. We cannot always have what we want.'[2]

On the one hand, in respect of personal goods and harms, a free society allows us the space to realize our individual desires and wants, provided they do not harm others (e.g. smoking). This is because we should seek to treat people as free agents ('ends in themselves'). And this goes to its logical conclusion for adults with mental capacity and of sound mind: we are free to refuse life-sustaining treatments without justification and to harm ourselves explicitly – even so far as suicide. These are freedoms or liberties (negative rights) writ large.

Positive rights or entitlements are different. These are things that society sees as good for anyone who is eligible and it obliges itself to provide the means for people to benefit from them. Collective goods come with duties of care. They involve others to facilitate, enable or implement. Healthcare is our example. Freedoms and entitlements are therefore different categories of rights. A move from one to the other changes it from, say, a harm that is tolerated to a potential good that should be offered and/or could be promoted. Indeed, it may become the preferred treatment on offer for certain people. Currently, suicide is tolerated but is actively limited by, for example, health promotion and the provision of helplines, and is considered to reflect grave distress or mental illness. This is the ethical reason why assisting suicide is categorically different from suicide. This impact is profound.

Legislating for changes in assisted suicide/euthanasia changes the category of suicide from a freedom to an entitlement for anyone who can make their case. This is a paradigm shift as it necessarily changes society's perception of life's intrinsic worth and exposes the complexity of our relationships as individuals within society. Assisted suicide/euthanasia demands the involvement of another moral agent, impacts the agent's autonomy and exposes the agent to moral hazards. There are few, if any, acts that will change a person as much as ending the life of another. Finally, if assisted suicide/euthanasia involves doctors, it introduces a new duty of care to end life in certain circumstances, with the personal and professional impact that ending a life entails.[15]

The language of clinicians who have written about their decision to assist suicide is emotive, insidious and subtle.[16] The literature that observes such decisions is revealing in speaking to the vulnerabilities of doctors of being in control.[6]

The view of the specialty

Lord Falconer's second bill of 2014 sought to legislate for physician-assisted suicide.[17] It was modelled on Oregonian legislation with the standard suite of 'safeguards'. To make an informed response, the APM surveyed its membership anonymously; 40% of members responded and the cross-section represented the APM's demographic. Legislation was opposed by 81.6%, but 11.8% thought the law should change; only 5% considered that medicine should be involved. In the independent Royal College of Physicians) survey of 2019, the palliative medicine cohort returned a similar result: 84% were opposed to physician-assisted suicide, 9% favoured legal change, but only 4.8% were willing to be involved directly.[18]

Returning to the 361 respondents in the APM survey, 16 (4%) were willing to prescribe lethal drugs; 79 (22%) were willing to prepare judgements about capacity, fixed will and any degree of coercion, and 256 (71%) were prepared to provide the court with factual data on diagnosis, extent of disease, the involvement of palliative care, etc. In terms of the effect on the delivery of palliative care, three respondents thought that physician-assisted suicide would have a very positive effect, 15 a positive effect and 80 had no view; 135 thought it would have an adverse effect and 128 a very adverse effect.[19]

Thematic analysis showed vulnerability, concerns over coercion and feelings of burden; the frailty of safeguards was a reason for opposition. In respect of the role of medicine and palliative care, duties of care, trust, the unsustainability of a clause allowing conscientious objection, disinvestment in care, reinforcement of the mythology around palliative care being euthanasia by the back door, and the negative impact on the specialty as a career choice were cited.[19]

Conclusion

 As palliative care physicians we have to think hard and rigorously about the ethical foundations of what we do in care as people die.

- We are clear that:
    - stopping treatments and suicide or physician-assisted suicide/euthanasia are not on a continuum as is often claimed;
    - there is no moral distinction between assisting suicide and administering euthanasia;
    - if assisted suicide/euthanasia is legal for anyone, unjustifiable discrimination will prevent its being confined for long to those with who have mental capacity and are dying, have life-limiting disease(s) and are adults, and it will ultimately extend to anyone who feels their life is no longer worth living.

- We are explicit about our motivations and intentions in offering, initiating or continuing treatments, balancing benefits and harms.

- Freedoms such as suicide and entitlements such as assisted suicide/euthanasia are different categories of rights. Moving a tolerated freedom to an entitlement means it should be offered to all and may become a preferred option for certain people. This impact is profound because it changes society's perception of life's intrinsic worth.

- Adding physician-assisted suicide/euthanasia as a treatment requires doctors to judge whether a life is harmful and consider or agree that a person would be better off dead. This conflict in duties is unsustainable.

There is still one question. Which is worse: not to kill someone who wants to die, or inadvertently kill someone who still wants to live? If society wants assisted suicide/euthanasia for its citizens, responsibility should be with the courts to decide and to instruct a named, trained operative outside healthcare to assist the suicide or administer euthanasia. This hermetic seal is the only way to protect patients from assisted suicide/euthanasia polluting their healthcare. Fewer than one in 20 palliative care physicians in the UK would be willing to perform physician-assisted suicide/euthanasia. Some support it in principle, which is entirely consistent with considering it incompatible with medicine, as they are separate questions.

References

1 Edwards MJJ. Opioids and benzodiazepines appear paradoxically to delay inevitable death after ventilator withdrawal. J Palliat Care 2005; 21: 299–302.

2 *Aintree University Hospitals NHS Foundation Trust v James* [2013] UKSC 67.

3 Seale C. End-of-life decisions in the UK involving medical practitioners. Palliat Med 2009; 23: 198–204.

4 George R. We must not deprive dying people of the most important protection. BMJ 2014; 349: g4311.

5 Kissane DW. The contribution of demoralization to end of life decision making. Hastings Cent Rep 2004; 34: 21–31.

6 Hicks MH. Physician-assisted suicide: a review of the literature concerning practical and clinical implications for UK doctors. BMC Fam Pract 2006; 7: 39.

7 Ganzini L, Goy ER, Dobscha SK. Prevalence of depression and anxiety in patients requesting physicians) aid in dying: cross sectional survey. BMJ 2008; 337: a1682.

8 Sleeman K, Chalmers I (2019). Assisted dying – restricting access to people with fewer than six months to live is discriminatory. Available from: https://blogs.bmj.com/bmj/2019/09/25/katherine-sleeman-and-iain-chalmers-assisted-dying%e2%81%a0-restricting-access-to-people-with-fewer-than-six-months-to-live-is-discriminatory/#disqus_thread (accessed 27 October 2019).

9 Vathorst SV. Concerning the basic idea that the wish to end suffering legitimates physician aid in dying for psychiatric patients. Am J Bioeth 2019; 19: 1–2.

10 Cook M (2019). US study says assisted suicide laws rife with dangers to people with disabilities. Available from: www.bioedge.org/bioethics/us-study-saysassisted-suicide-laws-rife-with-dangers-to-people-with-disabil/13245 (accessed 27 October 2019).

11 Association for Palliative Medicine of Great Britain and Ireland (2019). APM web materials on actively and intentionally ending life (variously called assisted suicide, assisted death, aid in dying and euthanasia). Available from: https://apmonline.org/news-events/apm-physician-assisted-dying-web-materials (accessed 27 October 2019).

12 Davies J, Willis D, George R The double effect is no doctrine, it's a reflective tool. Part 1. Eur J Palliat Care 2017; 24: 178–81.

13 George R, Regnard C. Lethal opioids or dangerous prescribers? Palliat Med 2007; 21: 77–80.

14 Walzer M. Just and unjust wars. 4th ed. New York: Basic Books, 2006.

15 MacLeod RD, Wilson DM, Malpas P. Assisted or hastened death: the healthcare practitioner's dilemma. Glob J Health Sci 2012; 4: 87–98.

16 Fraser G (2019). Right to die: interview with Canadian palliative care doctor Dr Sandy Buchman. Available from: www.holyrood.com/inside-politics/view,right-to-die-interview-with-canadian-palliative-care-doctor-dr-sandy-buchma_9904.htm (accessed 27 October 2019).

17 Assisted Dying Bill [HL] 2014–15. Available from: https://services.parliament.uk/bills/2014–15/assisteddying.html (accessed 27 October 2019).

18 Royal College of Physicians (2019). Assisted dying survey. Available from: www.rcplondon.ac.uk/projects/outputs/assisted-dying-survey-2019 (accessed 28 October 2019).

19 Association for Palliative Medicine of Great Britain and Northern Ireland. Doctors who care for dying people are unwilling to participate in physician assisted suicide. Available from: https://apmonline.org/wp-content/uploads/2019/01/press-release-apm-survey-confirms-opposition-to-physician-assisted-suicide-3.pdf (accessed 20 January 2020).

Chapter 8: Conclusions

Michael I. Bennett, Ruth E. Board, Penney Lewis, Peter Selby

The workshop and drafting of this publication have proved a challenging and productive exercise. We had four goals at the beginning of our workshop and for the preparation of this publication:

1   *To better inform members of the Association of Cancer Physicians (ACP) and the wider community about developments in choices in end of life care for cancer patients in the UK and internationally*

We believe that our workshop and this publication achieve this goal. The description of the current state of healthcare provision and legal position in the UK and internationally and the balanced representation of views about changes in the law in the UK should be an asset to all those involved in developing services and talking to patients and should perhaps inform the general social and political discussion.

2. *To be better able to answer questions from patients and respond to their requests, including questions about and requests for assisted dying in countries outside the UK*

Clinicians of all professions will be able to use the information provided about the legal status of a range of end of life decisions in different jurisdictions to help them individually in their decision taking and discussions with their patients and in training future healthcare professionals.

3. *To have a balanced and well-informed dialogue about choices available to patients in the UK and internationally, without developing a formal ACP position on change in UK law*

4. The feedback from the workshop suggests that we have achieved a balanced dialogue and avoided any attempts to reach a consensus about possible changes in the law. This was our purpose for two reasons: we knew that a comprehensive professional consensus was not possible at this time and that there were differing views across and within different professional groups in healthcare; also, we did not believe, and workshop participants did not believe, that healthcare professionals should slip into the error of believing that they are the ones who should take these vitally important social, legal and political decisions – their job is to be informed and engaged and to communicate effectively with patients and to practise within the limits of the current law.

To provide a basis of information for future educational activities

These articles will be made available electronically and widely disseminated through the ACP website (www.theacp.org.uk) and electronic library (http://ebook.ebnhealth.com). We welcome their use as an educational aid for discussions in small and large groups. We hope this professional educational exercise will also provide a useful educational base for a dialogue between patients, patient advocates and healthcare professionals that is active and ongoing. We can always improve the support we give to cancer patients as they face challenges at the end of life. We hope that this publication will be found to be informative, fair, balanced and worthwhile.

We venture to draw some conclusions. First, we emphasize that modern palliative care is a vital part of high-quality cancer care. It is a truly multi-professional healthcare activity. It draws on a wide range of technical skills including carrying out demanding interventions to relieve obstructions and perform minimally invasive nerve block procedures, and mastering the complex pharmacology of modern pain control and symptom relief. Moreover, the deployment of 'high tech) is always balanced by the judgement, grace and compassion that is essential for the best patient-centred palliative care practice. Any consideration of choices at the end of life for cancer patients must keep at its centre the need for equitable and ready access to the best palliative care. This is important to most cancer patients and it is the component of choice at the end of life that benefits most people.

There is an ongoing international trend towards widening choices for patients at the end of life to include assisted dying in some form. In jurisdictions where it is permitted, assisted dying seems to be the choice of a small proportion of patients at the end of their lives, most of whom are cancer patients. The introduction of an option for some form of assisted dying in many countries has been achieved through varied routes and has different characteristics in different jurisdictions. It does, however, appear feasible to introduce assisted dying into clinical practice without any evidence to date that it results in the deterioration of the provision of palliative care. There is some evidence in Canada that it may reinforce an interest in wide and equitable access to high-quality palliative care. Many countries have introduced measures to ensure that the interests and safety of young or vulnerable people are considered carefully and addressed, but it remains a challenging area. There is evidence that much public opinion in the UK supports some form of assisted dying. There is evidence that overall medical professional opinion in the UK is 'neutral) on this issue.

We do not see the comprehensive provision of high-quality palliative care and the introduction of assisted dying as alternatives in competition with each other. In some countries they already coexist and present choices for patients. The social, legal and political debate on legal change in the UK is likely to continue and we hope our workshop and publication will help healthcare professionals to contribute constructively to it.